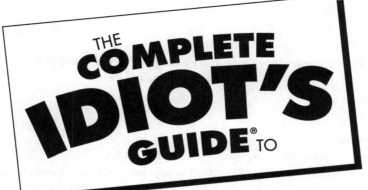

THE COMPLETE IDIOT'S GUIDE® TO

Weight Training

Illustrated

Third Edition

*by Deidre Johnson-Cane, Jonathan Cane, and
Joe Glickman*

ALPHA

A member of Penguin Group (USA) Inc.

To our families—who gave us the passion to lift and chutzpah to write.
—Deidre, Jonathan, and Joe

ALPHA BOOKS

Published by the Penguin Group

Penguin Group (USA) Inc., 375 Hudson Street, New York, New York 10014, USA

Penguin Group (Canada), 90 Eglinton Avenue East, Suite 700, Toronto, Ontario M4P 2Y3, Canada (a division of Pearson Penguin Canada Inc.)

Penguin Books Ltd., 80 Strand, London WC2R 0RL, England

Penguin Ireland, 25 St. Stephen's Green, Dublin 2, Ireland (a division of Penguin Books Ltd.)

Penguin Group (Australia), 250 Camberwell Road, Camberwell, Victoria 3124, Australia (a division of Pearson Australia Group Pty. Ltd.)

Penguin Books India Pvt. Ltd., 11 Community Centre, Panchsheel Park, New Delhi[md]110 017, India

Penguin Group (NZ), 67 Apollo Drive, Rosedale, North Shore, Auckland 1311, New Zealand (a division of Pearson New Zealand Ltd.)

Penguin Books (South Africa) (Pty.) Ltd., 24 Sturdee Avenue, Rosebank, Johannesburg 2196, South Africa

Penguin Books Ltd., Registered Offices: 80 Strand, London WC2R 0RL, England

Copyright © 2005 by Deidre Johnson-Cane and Jonathan Cane

International Standard Book Number: 978-1-59257-419-3
Library of Congress Catalog Card Number: 2005930933

10   8   7

Interpretation of the printing code: The rightmost number of the first series of numbers is the year of the book's printing; the rightmost number of the second series of numbers is the number of the book's printing. For example, a printing code of 05-1 shows that the first printing occurred in 2005.

Printed in the United States of America

Note: This publication contains the opinions and ideas of its authors. It is intended to provide helpful and informative material on the subject matter covered. It is sold with the understanding that the authors and publisher are not engaged in rendering professional services in the book. If the reader requires personal assistance or advice, a competent professional should be consulted.

The authors and publisher specifically disclaim any responsibility for any liability, loss, or risk, personal or otherwise, which is incurred as a consequence, directly or indirectly, of the use and application of any of the contents of this book.

Most Alpha books are available at special quantity discounts for bulk purchases for sales promotions, premiums, fund-raising, or educational use. Special books, or book excerpts, can also be created to fit specific needs.

For details, write: Special Markets, Alpha Books, 375 Hudson Street, New York, NY 10014.

Publisher: *Marie Butler-Knight*
Editorial Director: *Mike Sanders*
Senior Managing Editor: *Jennifer Bowles*
Development Editor: *Christy Wagner*
Senior Production Editor: *Billy Fields*
Copy Editor: *Jennifer Connolly*

Cartoonist: *Shannon Wheeler*
Cover/Book Designer: *Trina Wurst*
Photographer: *Peter Baiamonte*
Indexer: *Angie Bess*
Layout: *Becky Harmon*
Proofreading: *Donna Martin*

Contents at a Glance

Contents

Foreword

The sports world has changed dramatically over the past 30 years. In the early 1970s, sports were mainly restricted to male athletes on high school, college, and professional teams. With the passage of Title IX in 1972, the landscape of the sports world was forever changed. Women and girls of all ages now are as much a part of the sports world as men. For many reasons, social and health related, this evolution has been overwhelmingly positive.

Changes have not only been restricted to gender. The age of athletes has changed as well in the past 30 years. In today's sports world, the young athlete, often playing on competitive sports teams at 7 and 8 years of age, has created a new kind of sportsperson, such as the 10-year-old competitive soccer player. At the other end of the age spectrum, the elder athlete, the 80-year-old marathon runner and the 83-year-old swimmer, have defined new athletic possibilities for older Americans. In between, millions of Americans are running marathons, playing on basketball teams, and taking ballet class, all trying to stay fit and healthy.

With the landscape of the sports world changed, the field of sports medicine has changed as well. Sports medicine, the treatment and care of athletic individuals, has evolved with the changes in participant demographics. These include specific health programs designed for children, women, and the elderly. Each of these programs has the specific health needs of a particular group of athletes in mind.

Today's athletes require education and knowledge about preventive health to stay healthy, fit, and injury-free. This includes a whole spectrum of issues such as diet, sleep, exercise, and healthy lifestyle choices. Rather than fixing problems after they have been created, preventive health aims to educate athletes on how to avoid injuries before they occur.

For athletes, weight training is a major factor in the development and maintenance of healthy bones and muscles. In combination with proper diet and exercise, weight training is tremendously beneficial to athletes of all ages and at all stages of their careers. Recent studies have indicated that weight training, at any age, can reduce the likelihood of sports-related injury. Furthermore, weight training builds bone density, prevents osteoporosis, and is part of the preventive sports medicine knowledge with which every athlete should be familiar.

In my practice, weight-training discussions often start with the necessity of learning the proper technique to ensure safety and health. There are many stories from my office, as well as from many of my colleagues, where a well-intentioned athlete has injured him- or herself by trying to lift too much weight with improper technique. Learning the right way to lift makes a tremendous difference for both efficacy and safety.

The Complete Idiot's Guide to Weight Training Illustrated, now in its third edition, is part of the movement toward athletes educating themselves about the importance of preventive health. By learning proper technique, the do's and don'ts of weight training, the readers of this informative guidebook will learn volumes about how to do it the right way.

Use this book, make it part of your weight training practice, and most of all, enjoy your sports while keeping them healthy.

Best in health,

Jordan D. Metzl, M.D.

Jordan D. Metzl, M.D., is medical director of The Sports Medicine Institute for Young Athletes, Hospital for Special Surgery, New York, New York. A 17-time marathon runner and 2-time Ironman Triathlete, he is author of *The Young Athlete: A Sports Doctor's Complete Guide for Parents* (Little Brown, 2002).

Introduction

We've all seen the infomercials on TV where some model using the "Superduper Tummy Tuck" machine has achieved his statuesque body by supposedly using this gizmo for 20 minutes every other day. Never mind that the body-beautiful model is an out-of-work actor who has spent 3 hours a day working out for the last 10 years. The selling point behind virtually all these "quick-and-easy" fitness devices is that honing your body into a figure Michelangelo would be eager to sculpt is basically effortless. This, of course, isn't the case.

Getting into peak physical shape takes time and effort. That's the bad news. The good news is that you have plenty of time to realize the strong and supple physique you've always wanted. Why? Getting into and then staying in shape is a life-long process, and not something you do in frenetic preparation for your twentieth high school reunion or to look good at the beach. Done properly, strength training is an important piece in a process where you learn how to restore your body's natural gifts—gifts that are often stymied by our busy, modern lives.

While we can't guarantee that reading this book will turn you into the next governor of California, we feel quite confident that if you follow our advice and implement it correctly, you will look and feel better than you've ever felt before—it just might take longer than 20 minutes.

What You'll Find in This Book

This book is a complete guide to strength training, but it is also a primer on getting and staying in shape on a more comprehensive basis. We concentrate on lifting weights, but we hope to impress on you the importance of proper nutrition, posture, stretching, and cardiovascular exercise as well. Strength training will get you strong; implementing these other aspects will get you fit. We present you with everything the beginner needs to know to make his or her introduction to weight lifting as painless (literally and figuratively) as possible. You learn about everything from shopping for a gym to setting up your first exercise program to pushing through plateaus as you progress.

We've divided the book into three major parts:

In **Part 1, "Gearing Up,"** we fill you in on everything you need to know before you begin a weight-lifting program, including some important advice about how you really can't afford *not* to work out. Chapter 1 tells you all you need to know about choosing the right gym, and we also give you the lowdown on how to equip your home gym if that's the route you take. We also let you know about choosing the right duds for your workout. In Chapter 2, we move on to the basics of a proper diet as well as the pros and cons of the scores of nutritional supplements out there today. Chapter 3 addresses the dreaded, but often necessary, visit to the doctor as well as safety issues in the gym, while by Chapter 4, we move into the gym and begin stretching.

It's funny how many people who start lifting have little or no idea what muscles they're working. "I want to work these things," they say, pointing to their deltoids. That's where **Part 2, "The Workout,"** comes in. Chapter 5 gives you a rundown on what to expect when you begin lifting. We underscore the importance of proper form and technique—the foundation of any program. Chapters 6 through 12 are the guts of the how-to section. Each exercise is accompanied by photos and a thorough explanation of what to do.

Now that you've learned the nuances of the equipment, the exercises, and the philosophy behind working out, in **Part 3, "Leaner and Meaner,"** we show you how to put it all together. Chapter 13 gives you guidelines on which exercises to include in your routine depending on your goals and time constraints as well as what to do if things aren't working out the way you expected. Chapter 14 clues you in on some of the most common mistakes made by lifters and tells you how to avoid them. In Chapters 15 and 16, we introduce you to a variety of advanced techniques to help you take that next step. Chapter 17 gives you a primer on the basics of bodybuilding, powerlifting, and Olympic lifting—the three pillars in the pantheon of weight-lifting sports. In Chapter 18, we give the serious athlete and the weekend warrior suggested workouts to raise their game. In Chapter 19, you find everything you need to know about cardiovascular exercise, and in Chapter 20, we provide you with tips on how to fit all these great workouts into your busy schedule. Finally, Chapter 21 gives you a list of exercises you can do using resistance bands, for when you can't make it to the gym.

Extras

To make the learning experience as easy and as fun as possible, we've highlighted lots of tips and facts along the way. Look for the following elements throughout the book to guide you along:

Flex Facts

These sidebars are interesting tidbits and anecdotes. They're not essential for you to have a safe or effective workout, but you should find them informative and sometimes amusing.

Bar Talk

"Bar Talk" sidebars provide you with definitions of new terms introduced in the text. By adding them to your gymspeak vocabulary, you might not lift any better, but you will be better informed.

Spot Me

These are tips and pointers to help make your lifting more effective. Think of them as having a personal trainer giving you help throughout your workout. They highlight little things that might otherwise go unnoticed.

Weight a Minute

These sidebars highlight safety issues important to your health and welfare. The gym can be a dangerous and intimidating place if you don't know what to expect. Read these cautions carefully to ensure your workout is pain-free.

Acknowledgments

Writing a book is a little like building a beautiful body: it's a great idea with many rich rewards, but man, it boils down to plain old hard work. The three of us—friends when we started, better friends when we finished—enjoyed working on this project, but plenty of times we would rather have been doing something else. Of course, writing this book would have been far more difficult without the invaluable input of quite a few people.

Thanks to Ralph Anastasio of Printing House Fitness Center in New York City for the use of his great facility. Printing House is our favorite gym, and Ralph has been a constant supporter and friend.

Also, our models are more than just buffed bods and pretty faces—they're also all fine athletes and better friends. Special thanks to Susan Stanley, Laura Galbraith, Terrence Gerchberg, and Conrad Kiffin.

Special thanks from Deidre to her father and sister for their endless faith in her and to Laura Giovanella for her patience and support.

Jonathan would like to thank a few of his teachers—Bob Otto, John Wygand, Bob Perez, and Ralph Carpinelli—without whom this book would contain far fewer big words and sophisticated ideas. Thanks to his training mates for making him work, the athletes he coaches for keeping him honest, his co-authors for tolerating him, and most of all, his family for their support and patience.

Last, but not least, Joe wishes to thank his lovely, literate wife, Beth, and darling 9-year-old daughter, Willa. Most of all, he'd like to thank his co-authors, Jonathan, a terrible mountain biker but great coach, and "D," a beautiful woman who gets downright ugly when she wins World Powerlifting Championships. Without their wit and wisdom, he would still be wandering lost in the fitness forest.

Special Thanks to the Technical Reviewer

The Complete Idiot's Guide to Weight Training Illustrated was reviewed by an expert who double-checked the accuracy of what you'll learn here to help us ensure that this book gives you everything you need to know about weight training. Special thanks are extended to Dr. Bob Otto.

Dr. Robert M. Otto is professor and director of the Human Performance Laboratory at Adelphi University, Garden City, New York. He currently serves on the board of trustees of the American College of Sports Medicine. He has published and presented more than 200 papers on the role of exercise in health, disease, and functional performance. He is an avid triathlete and runner who has completed more than 80 triathlons and a dozen marathons.

Trademarks

All terms mentioned in this book that are known to be or are suspected of being trademarks or service marks have been appropriately capitalized. Alpha Books and Penguin Group (USA) Inc. cannot attest to the accuracy of this information. Use of a term in this book should not be regarded as affecting the validity of any trademark or service mark.

In This Part

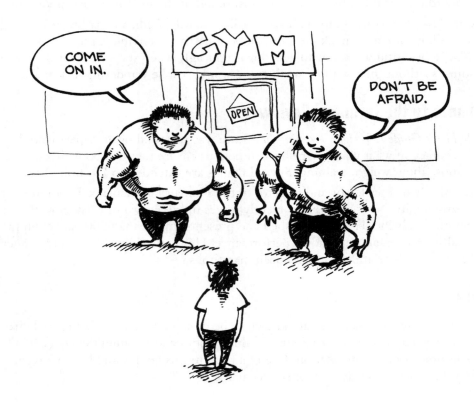

Part 1

Gearing Up

In this first part, we fill you in on everything you need to know before you begin a weight-lifting program, including some important advice about how you really can't afford *not* to work out. Many people want to work out but feel intimidated by the newness of this foreign place called a gym, full of sweaty strangers and loud music. In fact, a gym is a social place where you're likely to make good friends. In the following four chapters, we familiarize you with the nuances of the gym so those first days are largely anxiety-free.

In This Chapter

- ◆ Finding the gym for you
- ◆ Getting help: the lowdown on personal trainers
- ◆ Choosing home exercise equipment wisely
- ◆ Learning the ABCs of freeweights
- ◆ Dressing for success in the gym

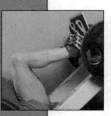
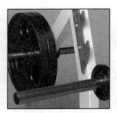
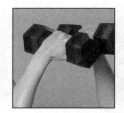
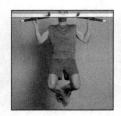
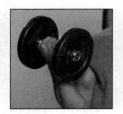
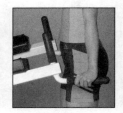

Look Before You Lift

There's a scene in an episode of *Seinfeld* in which a brassy, no-talent comedian tells Jerry he's gotten so big from lifting weights that his suits no longer fit him. "I'm huge!" he brags. "You really oughta lift," he instructs the slender Seinfeld. Jerry replies, "Why?" This basic bit of logic throws the "pumped" lifter for a loop. "Don't know," he says quizzically.

Actually, there are more good reasons to lift weights than there are good sitcoms on television. But before you leap into your workouts, it's important to take a look around the gym. In this chapter, we help you decide between working out at home or in a gym and give you tips on shopping for either. Plus we make sure you choose clothes that maximize both form and function. Read on!

Eenie, Meenie, Miney, Mo

Here's an obvious bit of advice that, oddly enough, takes many people by surprise: the more specific your fitness goals, the easier it is to pick a gym that suits your needs. In other words, are you just there to pump iron, or are you interested in taking aerobics classes, yoga, swimming, boxing, or playing basketball? Is taking a sauna a big plus or a big ho-hum? Remember, if your gym has these amenities and you choose not to use them, you're likely subsidizing someone else's use of them.

As long as we're on the obvious front: check to be sure the gym you join has hours that work for you. We know one gym in Brooklyn that sits over a synagogue and must close on the Sabbath as well as whenever there's a Jewish holiday. "Closed for the Ninth of Av? Never heard of that one!"

"Gosh," you may be saying, "I just want to find a gym and get in shape, not select a four-year college." Don't worry. In the pages that follow, we help you figure out what you should look for in an institution of higher fitness, factoring in everything from your legal rights to your creature comforts.

Neatness—or at Least Cleanliness—Counts!

Surveying a gym is a bit like looking for a home, only different. Instead of looking for closet space and listening for street noise, you want to focus on the general cleanliness of the gym area and locker rooms, as well as the quality of the equipment. When you enter a new gym for inspection, don your white gloves and prepare to judge!

Look for the following in the gym area:

◆ Take a good look at the general condition of the equipment. For example, are the cables you'll find on many pieces of gym equipment in good repair, or are they frayed?

◆ Check out the equipment's manufacturer. If it's Bodymaster, Cybex, Maxicam, or Nautilus, that's a good sign. Stu's, Herb's, or Skip's should send up a warning signal. Other reputable companies to look for are Hammer, Icarian, and Life Fitness.

◆ Is the upholstery covering the equipment worn and/or torn? If the equipment looks like the inside of a honky-tonk, you may consider your alternatives.

◆ Check out the dumbbells—the handheld weights you'll soon become familiar with. Are they the plated variety, which hold up well, or the hexagonal type that tend to bend and rust?

Now get yourself into the locker room and evaluate the following:

◆ Is the locker room clean?

◆ Are the lockers large enough to accommodate your gear? We've been to gyms where fitting your clothes into a skinny locker is like squeezing a thick English muffin into a narrow-slotted toaster. In winter, when you'll be toting even more clothes, this toaster phenomenon gets worse. So buyer beware.

◆ Are there lockers for rent? Renting a locker allows you to leave stuff at the gym, like a weight belt, shampoo, deodorant, or hair dryer—a lifesaver if you'll be heading for the office or the movies after your workout.

◆ Are the stalls in the bathroom clean? Or is the place like the restroom at an interstate rest stop? Is there toilet paper in the stall?

◆ Ditto for the shower stalls. A nice, hot, relaxing shower after a workout is supremely satisfying, unless the space is a moldy mess reserved for jungle explorers and cattle rustlers. Also, it's not a bad idea to check the water pressure. A dribbling showerhead just doesn't get it done.

◆ How about the upkeep of the steam room, sauna, and whirlpool? Again, these are excellent features—provided they're fit for human enjoyment.

Do You Have X, Y, and Z?

Gyms are a bit like restaurants: the basic product is the same, but the pomp and circumstance surrounding the workout/meal varies widely. To some, the only factors of concern when selecting a gym are (1) do they have enough equipment? and (2) is the price right? Everything else is window dressing.

Consider a musclehead gym we know in Brooklyn that's so austere and grungy it's almost cool. Inside, large, animated men with biceps the size of cantaloupes hoist prodigious amounts of freeweights like NFL linemen tossing back spare ribs. The grunting and groaning is so intense you'd almost think you were listening to natural childbirth. Shampoo and conditioner in the shower stalls? Get real! Patrons are lucky there's water in the water fountain. Nevertheless, the gym has 9 million pounds of freeweights, and the annual membership is about the cost of dinner for 9 at McDonald's. For some, that's just what the doctor ordered.

On the other hand, if you prefer a prettier setting, or if the sight of a spider in the bathroom sends you scurrying for a vaccination, you may want to consider a classier establishment.

Let's look at the amenities you may want to consider, realizing ahead of time that the more you get, the more you'll pay!

Ambience

Although you rarely hear the word *ambience* used to describe a gym, each establishment has its own feel, character, and mood. How do you feel when you enter a club? Are you comfortable there, or do you feel like racing out like a prisoner pardoned from jail? It's probably a good practice to trust your initial impression, because very often your gut-level feeling is what determines whether you stick with the place or not.

After working out in her neighborhood gym for many years, Deidre decided to join a gym that was closer to her job. Deidre appreciates the finer things in life but cares little if her gym has soft hankies in the ladies' room. However, the new club she joined had old, run-down equipment, a decrepit locker room, and played awful music really *loud!* Even for a tough gym-rat like her, the squalid scene detracted from the quality of her workouts. Before too long she was back in her bare-bones gym, which suddenly seemed much more pristine.

Know this: very few gyms let you tour their facility on your own. Usually, you'll be chaperoned by a salesperson whose job it is to get you to join. Keep this in mind, and don't let them rush you through a suspect area of the gym. In addition, don't let them hurry you into signing a contract on the spot if you're on the fence about whether to join or not. The salesperson might tell you the club is running a "special" sale, but more often than not, this select opportunity happens as frequently as a full moon—like every month! In other words, if you're not ready to buy, we assure you there will be another promotional deal sooner rather than later.

Curiously (or not), the same gym has a different feel depending on when you visit. Why? Gym regulars cycle through in predictable shifts: there's the prework crowd, the midmorning and afternoon lull set, the post-work rush, and the late-night revelers. That's why it's best to check out the gym you're examining at the hour you'll be working out. There's no sense in looking at a mellow, half-empty gym at noon if you're going to be rubbing elbows during peak evening hours with dozens of other patrons jockeying for the equipment.

If the place is too trendy or too low-rent, too loud or eerily silent for your tastes, or if the price is right but the neighborhood is wrong, remember you've got options. Be sure you check out one of the other 14,000-plus gyms out there. You're no doubt bound to find one that feels right for you.

Spot Me

For you web surfers, a great resource when shopping for a gym is www.healthclubs.com. Narrow your search by entering your zip code and what type of facilities you're looking for, and the site will instantly supply you with a list of gyms that fit your needs.

Bond or Bust

Here's a situation you may not have considered: on Monday you go to the gym to work your chest and back; on Wednesday you're back to do arms and shoulders when you learn that the gym is going belly up. Out of business. Chapter 11. Gone. Good-bye.

If the gym you join is bonded, you're guaranteed at least a partial refund. A bond is a contract between the state and the gym that provides, should the facility go out of business before the consumer's membership expires, the member will have some financial recourse. Roughly half of the states in the country require that a fitness center carry a bond of at least $50,000. If a bond is required in your state, the gym must have proof it has one should you ask. Again, if a bonded gym bites the dust, this doesn't mean you'll get a full refund, but it's insurance that you'll get at least some money back. If your gym is not bonded, there's not much you can do.

You might think calling your state's chamber of commerce or Better Business Bureau to see if your gym has a bond might seem like overkill, but gyms go out of business all the time, and sometimes under shady circumstances. Deidre once worked as a massage therapist at a health club that one day just closed its doors as suddenly as a three-card monte dealer folds his cardboard table. Even worse, in the days preceding this unannounced event, the owners offered tremendous deals on multiyear memberships. Obviously, these guys were trying to rake in as much cash as possible before closing up shop. (The only recourse any member had was to break in and hock the furniture. Try selling a used leg extension machine on the street—it's not a pretty sight.)

Your Escape Clause

You've got another good reason to read your gym contract carefully before you sign. Most states provide some sort of "buyer's remorse" clause in the contract that gives you anywhere from 24 to 72 hours to cancel your membership without being penalized. Similarly, there may be a clause in the contract to cover you if you move out of the area or are injured before your contract runs out. Some gyms allow members to "freeze" their memberships for certain periods—after having a baby, after being injured, to take a long vacation, and so on. And often if you move a significant distance from your gym (usually 25 miles), you'll be entitled to a prorated refund.

We realize you didn't buy this book to read about contracts, but know this: you can often have riders added to your contract. Remember that smiling salespeople often have more flexibility in what they can offer than they let on. You might be able to negotiate a family membership deal or a group discount if you recruit new members. If the gym doesn't offer discounts, you may be able to add another month on your membership or have a personal training session tossed in the mix. Remember, if you don't ask, you'll never know what accommodations you may be able to obtain.

For example, if you regularly travel out of town for weeks or months at a time, you can probably have the contract amended to account for this. Alternatively, your club might be affiliated with a national chain or organization (IHRSA, the International Health, Racquet and Sportsclub Association, is the largest and most reputable) that allows you to work out at another gym while you're on the road—usually free or at a discounted rate.

Just How Much Is This Going to Cost?

Pick a number between $99 and $9,999, and you've narrowed the price of joining a gym. In other words, the cost of a health club membership can vary widely, even within the same gym, because there are peak and off-peak memberships, month-to-month or annual contracts, and several options in between.

What's this about a month-to-month contract, you ask? Well, most clubs offer them, and they have several advantages over an annual contract:

- You won't have to lay out a lot of cash when you join.
- If you're not comfortable with the gym, just finish out the month, and you won't feel a financial pinch.
- Ditto if you move, travel a lot, get injured, or are abducted by aliens

But there's always another side of the coin, isn't there? Here are some of the disadvantages of having a month-to-month contract:

- If you continue to work out, it will end up costing you more at the end of the year.
- There's usually an "initiation fee" associated with month-to-month memberships that is often waived or nonexistent with annuals.

Give Me Exercise, or Give Me Death

Okay, we said we were done talking about your gym contract, but we think you should know a few more things. Here's an incident that illustrates a bogus practice employed by a gym in Brooklyn. This particular club allows you to pay on a monthly basis by automatically deducting the fee from your checking account. However, when a patron we know wanted to quit, she had to mail a certified letter. Then the gym could charge her another monthly fee until 30 days after it received the letter. In short, they made getting out of the contract as easy as settling a debt with the Mafia. Protect yourself by familiarizing yourself with the club's policy on cancellations. Many require 30 to 60 days' written notice.

As a consumer, you have rights when you purchase a membership from a health club.

(Remember that the contract not only spells out your commitment to the gym, but it also protects you against fraudulent acts by the owners.) In fact, most states have specific statutes that spell out consumers' rights when it comes to health clubs.

That said, we don't mean to imply that every gym—or even most gyms—is out to rook you. Far from it. Most gyms are legitimate businesses that make a profit by providing good service. But as in all things, when it comes to signing on the dotted line and handing over a check—buyer beware!

Evaluating the Trainers

Trainers present yet another one of those good news/bad news deals. The well-trained, knowledgeable, concerned fitness expert is an invaluable asset in the gym. They can help motivate you, offer advice on everything from nutrition to stretching, and help guide you through your workout. If you've got the will—and sometimes even if you don't—a good trainer has the way. The bad news, however, is that the staff at many fitness centers isn't always well trained, informed, or concerned.

Depending on a trainer's qualifications, reputation, and demand, expect to pay anywhere from $25 to $100 an hour for a training session. (Introductory sessions are often available to new members.) Some trainers trim the price if you work with a partner.

Keep in mind that anyone who walks and talks can call himself a "personal trainer," "exercise physiologist," or "fitness instructor." Scary as it sounds, in most states you need a license to cut hair but not to be a personal trainer.

The better establishments are staffed with trainers who have graduate degrees in exercise physiology, biomechanics, or other health sciences. In others, the instructors may have no laurels to rest on other than their beefy pectoral muscles. In-house certifications offered by some of the big national chains are as tough to pass as basket weaving. Essentially, their requirements are minimal, and the certification is just a way to let the gym tell folks that its staff is certified.

Weight a Minute

Don't be impressed just because a trainer is "certified." Clubs often have their own certifications—usually just a gimmick to pump up the appearance of their staff's credentials.

It's a good idea to check with the salespeople about the staff's qualifications. Scores of alphabet-soup certifications exist. The most respected is the American College of Sports Medicine (ACSM), although other organizations, such as the National Strength and Conditioning Association (NSCA) and the American Council on Exercise (ACE), also have certification programs.

If you do opt to work with a trainer, even for a few sessions to help you get started, be sure your trainer is not only qualified but insured as well. We sincerely hope it never happens, but if you are injured due to a trainer's neglect, you'll want your trainer to have liability insurance.

Now that you've had a chance to evaluate the idea of making a gym a part of your life, let's take a look at another viable option: creating a home gym that works for you.

There's No Place Like Home

Okay, let's say you're starting to think that working out at home is the way to go for you. What now? Well, now you've got to look into the future a bit and anticipate some of the challenges you may face. Don't worry, we'll walk you through it!

One important disadvantage of working out at home is that you have no spotter, a kind soul who will be sure you don't drop a weight on your head. Most home gym equipment is designed to minimize (and/or eliminate) this problem, but the potential still exists. Let's take a look.

Recognizing and Avoiding Home-Gym Pitfalls

It sounds perfect, doesn't it? If you have gym equipment at home, you can work out in privacy on your own schedule. No driving to the gym, no waiting for equipment, no need to worry about closing time. What could be better?

Before you assume home is where the exercise is, consider a few built-in pitfalls. Perhaps the most important one concerns safety—an issue we'll return to again and again throughout this book. If you're working out at home, you're almost always also working out alone, and that can be dangerous.

For instance, one day many moons ago, Joe came home and found his father stuck upside down like a bat hanging helplessly in a pair of inversion boots (an odd but once-popular piece of home gym equipment). One can only imagine what this poor old man would have done had no one come along to extricate him from his perilous predicament. Another time, Mr. Glickman was benching a modest amount of weight and was unable to press the bar from his chest. Stuck like a mouse in a trap, he slowly, painfully, rolled the weight toward his knees until he was able to squeeze out from below. Although these examples are humorous, each year 5 to 12 deaths are reported from weight training. Usually the cause of death is suffocation from dropping the bar across the neck during the bench press. These kinds of stories are virtually nonexistent in a gym, where patrons and trainers typically rush to your assistance.

Needless to say, because you are alone you need to take extra care to read the instructions that come with your home unit. If there's anything you don't understand, don't hesitate to call the manufacturer. Many units come with a video. Take the time to watch it—it could spare you an injury.

What You Need and What It Costs

Assuming you're like us and plan on working out until you're put out to pasture, setting up a home gym is more economical over the long term. (Actually, working out in a pasture is rather appealing as well!) Of course, if your shiny, high-tech piece of equipment becomes the featured item in a garage sale, you've been penny-wise and weight-foolish. Let's examine the cost of a complete home gym. We'll start with the equipment, which should include these three components:

- ◆ *Cardiovascular* **equipment.** You need some type of machine—stationary bike, rowing machine, or treadmill—that gets your ticker ticking.
- ◆ **Resistance equipment.** This apparatus helps you build muscle.
- ◆ **An exercise mat.** We discuss stretching at length in Chapter 12, but for now, know that working on your flexibility should be an integral part of any fitness regimen. A mat makes stretching and abdominal exercises far more comfortable.

Bar Talk

Cardiovascular exercise is any activity that elevates your heart rate over a sustained period of time. Your body's cardiovascular system includes your heart and lungs.

Cardio Action

What type of cardio machine should you buy? And how much can you expect to spend? Let's do a little imaginary shopping.

A stationary bike with bells and whistles like the LifeCycle can cost as much as $2,000, or you can spend as little as $300 for a basic stationary model. Here's the catch-22: if you're not sure you'll use it, it's best to start with the cheaper model. If, however, you're planning to become the next Lance Armstrong, the sturdier machine is preferable. Years ago, one of Jonathan's future teammates on his cycling team, a guy who hadn't cycled or exercised in years, started riding on a low-rent stationary bike he bought for a song. Before long, he had ridden it so often he ground it into pencil shavings. Afterward, he started riding on the road and went on to become one of the best riders in the state. If you already have a bicycle, a fine way to work out indoors is to buy a contraption that allows you to remove the front wheel and ride your bike indoors. State-of-the art models can go for as much as $1,500, but usually, such an apparatus goes for between $100 and $250.

If biking isn't your thing, let your feet do the walking and buy a treadmill. As is true for the stationary bike, you have a whole range of options for a treadmill, ranging in price from $500 to $5,000. Again, if you're going to use it regularly, it's far better to drop four figures on a solid machine. Three brands we particularly like are Star Trac, Life Fitness, and Precor.

Don't like to run or bike? A variety of other machines help get your heart pumping, including the Concept II rowing machine, NordicTrack cross-country ski simulators, stair climbers like the StairMaster, and the increasingly popular elliptical trainers that provide a great, low-impact workout.

The Weight Stuff

Now that we've explored the world of cardio equipment, it's time to discuss the meat and potatoes (or better yet, the broiled fish and brown rice, but we'll get to the diet stuff later in the book!) of the home gym: resistance equipment.

Here's what you should look for in an "all-in-one" unit:

- **A variety of exercises.** No matter how effective the exercise, a continuing routine of the same few exercises will leave you feeling bored.

- **Ease of movement from one exercise to another.** If transitioning from one exercise to another is difficult or time-consuming, you're not likely to use the machine. Or if you do use it, you're not likely to get a good workout.

- **Enough resistance to grow with you as you get stronger**. Right now, the lightest weight on the machine may be just a little too heavy for you to lift, but—as hard as it may be to imagine now—you won't be in that position for long. You'll get stronger and stronger, and you'll want a machine that will help you do just that. If you have to do 38 repetitions of an exercise to tax yourself, you need to increase the weight.

- **An objective measure of your progress.** You need a way to tell how strong you're getting from one week to the next. Progress is inspirational. If you see that you're able to do 10 more repetitions of a particular exercise, you're more likely to keep at it.

Quite a few multifunction strength-training machines on the market are versatile, sturdy, and safe. Of course, each has its advantages and disadvantages. Three of the best-selling and most effective units are the Total Gym (in

which you slide a sled and your body weight through a variety of exercises, adjusting the angle to change the resistance), the Soloflex (which uses elastic bands for resistance), and our personal favorite, the Bowflex (which uses patented "Power Rods" for resistance). Other home-gym, multifunction options come from Universal, Weider, Parabody, and Paramount.

The Power of Freeweights

If newfangled ideas like rubber bands and Power Rods don't do it for you, you can buy an adjustable bench ($300 to $500) and a set of freeweights, and knock yourself out (but not literally!). Although initially this might seem like the simpler, less-expensive way to go, the costs quickly add up, and it can become far more expensive than you anticipated. Furthermore, for the novice, the use of freeweights in an unsupervised setting makes us more than a wee bit nervous. Still, a freeweight setup at home can work quite well if you take the time to learn the rules and then follow them.

Now for the cost. Unless you're training to be the next governor of California, you probably don't want or need a full set of dumbbells in your home. A good option is a pair of adjustable dumbbells such as the PowerBlock. Selling for roughly $200, the PowerBlock enables you to easily and quickly adjust the weight of the barbell from 5 to 45 pounds. Newcomers in the adjustable dumbbell field include Probell and Versabell, each of which offers similar features.

When shopping for a bar and weights (also known as plates), you have a few options. "Olympic" bars, found in just about every gym, are 7 feet long and weigh 45 pounds. (Shorter, lighter bars are also available.)

Plates are available in 2.5- through 100-pound increments. Figure on spending about 25¢ per pound—a sum that adds up if you're a budding moose. Throw on a pair of collars (the clips that secure the plates at either end of the bar), and you're good to go for just about any of the exercises we describe in future chapters. We say "just about" because a few are unsafe to do without a spotter. We note which the risky ones are so you don't end up with an imprint of a barbell on your nose.

As we've said, unless you're willing to spend a small fortune, you'll never duplicate the wide range of equipment a good gym can offer (to say nothing of the guidance trainers can provide). However, even the best gym in the solar system does you no good if you don't use it. Working out in a gym is the most reliable way to build a fitter body, but a home gym is certainly the next best thing.

Strain in Style

What you wear to the gym is an issue of the utmost importance that really doesn't matter. By that we mean if it's comfortable, allows a full range of motion, and adheres to gym regulations, you could wear a tuxedo with tails or an evening gown and be good to go. This sounds ridiculous—and it is—but a few years ago, a terrific runner ran the New York City Marathon in a tuxedo jacket and shorts. (He discarded the black shoes and went with a pair of Nikes.)

So while you could work out effectively in a burlap bag, what you wear is of enormous personal relevance to who you are and what kind of statement you want to make—if you want to make any at all. Are you flashy or modest? A Lycra proponent or fan of organic cotton? Do you go with the neon lime green bike jersey and large silver hoop earrings or stick with the ripped T-shirt you wore when you went fishing with your Uncle Sylvester? In this section, we outline your options and make some recommendations about the workout clothes that might be right for you.

Do Clothes Make the Athlete?

Although we adhere to the philosophy of "to each his own," some people's workout attire can be perplexing. Deidre and Joe frequently find themselves working out next to a hulking guy who can lift a compact car and the kitchen sink. However, no matter how hot it gets, he wears an XXL sweatshirt and long baggy pants. Although he has the body of an NFL linebacker, the self-effacing chap refuses to show skin. Another full-bodied woman they know wears skintight outfits that would make Beyoncé blush.

Even more confusing is the dignified gent who works out in the same immaculate outfit every time: red tank top, blue shorts, white socks, and white sneakers. This is a perfectly fine outfit, but we're dying to know if he has two dozen of the same items (and if so, why?); and, if he has just one of each, does that mean he's laundering them after every workout? These, dear reader, are some of the questions that can weigh on a petty man's mind.

Simply put, picking an outfit to exercise in at the gym can be purely perfunctory or a fair bit of fun. We have more than a few biases on the subject we'll gladly share with you in the following pages, but the bottom line is: if the garment fits, wear it.

The Threads

The best workout clothing consists of any combination of comfortable garments that allow freedom of movement and a modicum of modesty. When Joe began competing in kayak marathons with international paddlers, he was initially surprised to see that the majority of the world-class Australian and South African kayakers he raced against wore baggy T-shirts while the Americans often wore tight tank tops. Why the baggy look? These guys had chiseled upper bodies straight from central casting. It's comfortable, mate! In other words, if you've got the goods, why compromise comfort for vanity? Before you could say rip curl, many of the Americans started wearing extra-large as well.

Here's a basic list of acceptable gym threads:

- Sweatpants
- Shorts
- Leggings
- T-shirts
- Tank tops
- Sports bras
- Sweatshirts

Although some people find wearing a tank top too revealing, keep in mind that it's always a good idea to concentrate on the muscle groups you're working, so if you're concentrating on your upper body, a tank top may be just the thing. Not only is it easier to focus on the task at hand if you can see the muscle actually lengthening and contracting, it can also be a good motivational tool to see your muscles grow before your eyes—a phenomenon known as the *pump*.

> **Bar Talk**
>
> Lifters often refer to the swelling in a muscle immediately after lifting as the **pump**. Although it appears that the muscle is growing as you lift, what you see is actually the muscle becoming temporarily engorged with blood—not the same thing as when the muscles themselves grow.

When working her upper body, Deidre usually wears a sports bra and sweatpants, and she dons a T-shirt and shorts when she works her lower body.

Joe, who has arguably the largest collection of race T-shirts in North America, tends to modify his attire according to the aerobic activity he's doing that day. If he's going to run and lift, he wears jogging shorts and brings along an extra T-shirt (no problem there). If he's going to cycle or use the Concept II rower, he's likely to wear bike shorts, and, you guessed it, a T-shirt. Also, on "leg" day, he prefers bike shorts because they offer better support when he does squats.

Jonathan, the triathlon coach who has been known to dine in trendy Manhattan restaurants in a black warm-up suit (arguing that, strictly speaking, it *is* a suit), doesn't really care what he's wearing as long as he's working out. In fact, Jonathan probably would lift in a lobster bib if he forgot to pack one of his 9 million T-shirts.

Women's Wear

Since the 1980s, more and more women have begun flocking to the gym. In the early days, it seemed as if women were wary of "looking like men" and overemphasized their femininity in their dress instead of focusing on the fact that they were athletes working out. This may (or may not) explain the popularity of the thong that scores of women wore to the gym.

In case you missed it, the thong is a one-piece leotard cut extremely high on the hips with a thin strip of cloth wedged uncomfortably between the buttocks. In gym parlance, it is known as *butt floss*. Many women looked downright sexy in the thing, but it had to be one of the cruelest fashion hoaxes this side of platform shoes, because essentially you were walking around with a self-imposed wedgie.

Luckily, these days the thong is mostly a collector's item packed neatly beside collections of *Jane Fonda's Greatest Aerobic Hits*. Today, most women who exercise regularly wear a sports bra and T-shirt with sweats or shorts.

If you do go the sports bra route and are amply endowed, be sure you can jog and/or take an aerobics class without doing yourself bodily harm. Similarly, causing a traffic accident might be good for your ego, but it could be bad for your conscience.

The Treads

If you hadn't already noticed, a trip to a well-equipped sporting goods store will reveal just how specialized workout gear has become. This is especially true in the footwear realm. In fact, never-throw-out-a-pair-of-running-shoes jocks like Jonathan and Joe each have at least 44 pairs. (Okay, maybe more, but we don't have the time to tally them all.) Think we're exaggerating? Here's a basic outline of the footwear you could find in our collective closets:

◆ Running shoes for the road (lots of them!)

◆ Trail running shoes

◆ Cycling shoes for biking on the road

◆ Cycling shoes for mountain biking and touring

◆ Basketball shoes

◆ Tennis shoes

◆ Cross-training shoes (hybrid sneakers designed to do a bit of everything)

◆ Water shoes (slipperlike footwear designed for kayakers)

◆ Approach shoes designed for easy hiking

◆ Sports sandals

Spot Me

When buying a new pair of shoes, it's a good idea to try them on in the evening, because your feet tend to swell toward the end of the day. What feels good at 9 A.M. might be a wee bit snug at dinnertime.

With the obvious exception of cycling shoes that feature protruding cleats that leave you walking like a petrified tree, most of the previously mentioned footwear is fine for just lifting weights. Remember that there have been many Olympic-level marathon runners who ran like the wind barefoot. So although the sport specificity in footwear does have its place, you can wear just about anything as long as it fits and gives you adequate support.

Herein lies the rub. Ideally, your footwear should provide you with ample arch support as well as proper medial (inside aspect of the foot) and lateral (outside) support. If you've ever had any foot pain, your best bet is to go to a store known for its sneaker savvy. Be specific with the salesperson about what you'll be doing in these sneakers. If you know you're *flat-footed* (have no arch), *overpronate* (walk on the inner portion of your foot), or *supinate* (walk on the outer portion), inform the salesperson; if he knows what he's doing, he should recommend shoes designed for those specific conditions. If you don't understand pronation, buy whatever feels best and, over time, monitor where the majority of the wear and tear on your footwear occurs. (If you're a runner, this will quickly become obvious.) Generally speaking, when you're weight lifting, a cross-training shoe would be your best bet for appropriate support.

Bar Talk

To **overpronate**, as it relates to walking, is to bear most of your weight on the inner portion of your foot. You can often tell by looking at the wear pattern on the soles of your shoes whether you pronate or **supinate**, which means to bear weight on the outer portion of your foot as you walk. To have a **flat foot** (*pes planus*) means to be without arches.

Don't Mention It

If ever there were a perfect place to discuss the ins and outs of sports bras, here it is. The three things to remember are proper fit, comfort, and structure.

◆ **Fit.** When shopping for a sports bra, always try it on before you get to the gym. Once you've got it on, clap your hands overhead; if the plastic band moves up your chest, it's too tight. You don't want to start working out and discover you're wearing an iron corset that doesn't allow you to breathe. And you don't want to fret about peek-a-boo bosom while you're lying in the middle of a bench or performing another cleavage-revealing exercise.

◆ **Comfort.** To continue on our sartorial theme: looking good doesn't equal feeling good. Besides, the better you feel when you work out, the more apt you are to keep training!

◆ **Structure.** Basically, you have two choices in sports bras: compression and encapsulation. Neither sounds terribly forgiving, but the latter tends to be the most comfortable. True to its name, the compression bra presses (read: squishes) the breasts against the chest in a single mass. This style is more appropriate for small- to medium-breasted women. Like a brassiere, the encapsulation type is built to hold each breast in a cup. This works better for full-figured women.

Wrap It Up

One of the neat things about strength training is that you can do it in a sophisticated gym with high-tech equipment or in a bare-bones basement with a bench, a few handheld weights, and plenty of desire. In either setting, however, you can bring nothing more than what you're wearing or an assortment of goodies that may (or may not) help you get stronger.

We're talking about weight belts, wrist and knee wraps, and gloves. Is this stuff necessary? Not really. Can the mere sight of this equipment get you psyched to go to the gym? Could be. Let's talk a bit about each one, and you can decide for yourself.

Buckle Up!

To belt or not to belt, that's a question that has generated a fair bit of debate among fitness devotees. The good news is that wearing a *weight belt* reminds you to maintain erect posture while you lift. The bad news is twofold: the belt offers support to the muscles in your lower back and abdomen that you're trying to strengthen, and wearing one can give you a false sense of security that may have you trying to lift more weight than is safe or necessary. Of course, if you have a weak lower back, a belt may be necessary to work out pain-free until we can help strengthen your abdominal and lower back muscles.

Bar Talk

A **weight belt** is made from thick, dense leather and is roughly 6 inches wide. It's buckled securely around your waist just above your hips.

In many ways, wearing a belt offers more psychological comfort than actual aid. If you suffer from low-level chronic back pain, wearing one can be comforting—it's like a heating pad without the heat, if you will. Furthermore, it's like an athlete who rubs the head of the trusty old trainer before taking the field. As they approach an imposing bar loaded with weight, many lifters cinch the buckle one notch tighter, a gesture that gets them psyched for the challenge more than anything else.

During her powerlifting days, Deidre wore a belt. But remember, her sport was about demonstrating strength; your goal in the gym is to gain strength. In other words, her goal was to lift the heaviest weight she possibly could, so wearing a belt while she squatted or deadlifted helped to up her totals. Again, we're concerned about what your muscles can do, not what your gear can do. Unless you feel you need to wear a belt, we recommend you don't.

For a belt to offer any significant support, it has to be pulled so tight you'd barely be able to whistle. By comparison, the corsets worn by female French nobility were as comfy as housedresses. In fact, before Deidre would approach a *squat* or deadlift, it would take two strong people to yank on her belt to get it tight enough to give her sufficient support. Hauling a marlin into a fishing boat wasn't as much of a struggle.

Bar Talk

The **squat** is a great full-body exercise that involves performing a deep knee-bend with a barbell across your back. Sounds intimidating, but fret not; we take you through the proper execution of this movement in Chapter 7.

It's a Wrap

You can use two kinds of wraps in the gym: wrist wraps and knee wraps. Wrist wraps are shorter and affixed with Velcro, while the longer knee wraps are cinched by tucking the wrap under itself and pulling.

Remember, for wraps to be effective, they have to be pulled pretty tight. There are only a few good reasons to wear wrist wraps:

◆ If you've recently suffered a wrist injury and need the support.

◆ If you have a tendency to *hyperextend* your wrists while you perform a bench press, it's a good idea to wrap. Otherwise, you could drop the bar.

Bar Talk

To **hyperextend** means to bend a body part beyond its normal anatomical or neutral position. For example, if you straighten your arm to lock your elbow, it will end up in a straight line. People who are called "double-jointed" can lock their elbow beyond that straight-line position so it looks as though their elbow is bending in the opposite direction. This is called hyperextension of your elbow.

Knee wraps? We're generally against them. These mummifying wraps are usually worn to support you when you're performing squats or using the leg press or leg extension machine. (For descriptions of these exercises, see Chapter 7.) We don't like knee wraps for the same reason we're generally against weight belts. Unless you're squatting or pressing a ton of weight, a person with healthy knees who wears them is wasting his or her time. Or worse.

The reason one does these exercises in the first place is to strengthen the muscles around the knee joint. When you wrap your knees, you remove a significant amount of the workload from the muscles and transfer it to the wraps. Simply put, wearing knee wraps defeats the purpose of the exercise.

Here's where people get confused. Wearing wraps helps you lift more weight, which should be good, right? Wrong! Being able to lift more weight is only good if it comes as the result of your muscles getting stronger, not because you've fortified yourself with wraps.

This "might makes right" logic highlights an important point: your lifting should be about getting strong, not seeming strong. This move-as-much-weight-as-possible syndrome, which afflicts men far more than it does women, is counterproductive to health and is as misguided as erecting an ornate roof before you've built a sound foundation.

We can hear the dissenters saying, "If I lift more with the wraps, my leg muscles won't get injured, and I'll get stronger faster." Nice try. Just because your securely wrapped knees can handle an increased load doesn't mean your back or other body parts can. So ironically, wrapping your knees to protect this complex and vulnerable joint may actually end up jeopardizing your safety rather than ensuring it.

Finger Wraps

A noncontroversial option in the lifting game is the wearing of gloves. Weight-lifting gloves, which typically cost around $10, have padded palms and cut-off fingers for ventilation and dexterity. Gloves are good if you look at calluses with disdain, and they can come in handy during certain abusive exercises such as chin-ups and lat pull-downs, which you'll read more about in later chapters.

When Deidre started lifting 10 years ago, she used gloves until she realized that her feel for the weight improved without them. What does "feel for the weight" mean? Many experienced lifters feel that the greater the contact they have with the bar, the easier it is to lift the weight. Try both and see for yourself.

Like Deidre, Jonathan and Joe go gloveless. A kayaker whose hands are usually callused and cracked from gripping a paddle hours a day in saltwater, Joe finds that the calluses he's built from lifting help fortify his mitts while paddling.

If you decide to don gloves, try to find a pair that have a grippy texture on the palms, and be sure they fit your hands snugly without restricting your movement.

Pads

Instead of gloves, some folks prefer pads, which are small, flat, neoprene squares that are held in your palms like mini-potholders. Not only do they offer the same comfort and improved grip as gloves, but you also won't have to worry about sweaty-palm syndrome. The downside is that because you have to carry them around, they tend to disappear like socks in a dryer. Jonathan has collected enough pads from his gym's lost and found to tile Madison Square Garden.

Straps

Straps are another common piece of paraphernalia you'll see in the gym. Made of sturdy, nonstretch material, straps are worn around your wrists and then wrapped around the bar you plan to lift. The purpose of straps is to ease the burden on the gripping muscles in your hands and forearms that often fatigue before the larger working muscles.

Take exercises such as deadlifts, pull-ups, and cable rows, which we'll explain in depth in Chapter 8. These exercises all involve movements that tax large muscles and hence require you to lift a fair bit of weight. Overusing straps can prevent those hand and forearm muscles from becoming stronger, but they are useful when a weak grip inhibits you from completing the exercise, a common occurrence if you're lifting a lot of weight.

As you may have gathered by now, we're not big proponents of gadgets that make your exercises easier. Still, after you spend enough time at the gym, you'll see tremendously strong people who lift with a weight belt, wrist and knee straps, and gloves. What's up with that?

People who lift a lot often have developed their own habits—good and bad—over many years of experimentation. However, when you start out, it's important to establish good habits, to lift with sound technique and with as little interference as possible—just you, the weight, knowledge, and plenty of desire.

The Least You Need to Know

◆ A good gym is the sum total of its parts. Know what to look for, and you won't regret your choice.

◆ Not all trainers are created equal. Learn which degrees are worth more than the paper they're printed on.

◆ Setting up a home gym may be more cost effective than paying a gym membership— assuming you use it.

◆ Your workout gear should look good and feel better.

◆ When buying shoes, let fit and function be your guide.

◆ Weight belts, wrist and knee wraps, and gloves can help or hinder you. Use them with care.

In This Chapter

- ◆ Eating: what and when
- ◆ Weighing the pros and cons of protein
- ◆ Losing weight without dieting
- ◆ Understanding how supplements may do more harm than good
- ◆ Learning the truth about supplements
- ◆ Using coffee to boost energy and performance

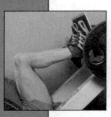 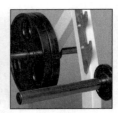 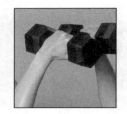 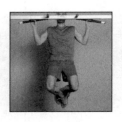 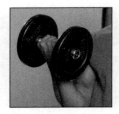 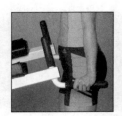

Chapter 2

Food for Thought

Ask any bodybuilder, triathlete, or racehorse trainer about the importance of proper nutrition, and he's likely to say the same thing: you are what you eat.

Sure, lifting can (and should) be an important part of your fitness regimen, but if you neglect proper nutrition, you're likely to sabotage your potential gains in the gym as well as your overall health. We all know people who seem to flourish while eating a diet of pastrami sandwiches, jelly donuts, and milkshakes, but most people pay a steep price for such gluttony.

Typically, if you neglect your diet, you're destined to struggle with your weight, feel sluggish during the day, or worse, invite sickness and disease. Even if you exercise regularly and have a washboard stomach, ignoring sound nutrition means you'll probably struggle through your workout. "I just didn't have it today" is a common complaint heard in the gym. It says a great deal about the individual's body chemistry and the lack of the fuel it needs to function.

As you probably know, enough myths and misinformation about nutrition are floating around out there to confuse even the most knowledgeable doctor. Don't despair. In this chapter, we walk you through this dietary quagmire and explain what constitutes a sensible diet. We also discuss the changes you may need to make as you improve your fitness level and health. If you have less body fat than an underfed marathoner, have more energy than a nuclear power plant, and eat plenty of fresh vegetables and lean protein, you probably should just skip to the next chapter. If not, grab a pen or pencil, and let's get shopping.

How Much Is Just Enough?

Let's start at the beginning—the basics of a sensible diet for the average healthy adult.

According to the U.S. Department of Agriculture (USDA), the "standard" healthy male weighs 154 pounds, and his female counterpart tips the scales at 121. The phrase we often hear—Recommended Dietary Allowances (RDA) or Recommended Daily Intake (RDI)—refers to the levels of protein, vitamin, and mineral intake considered adequate to meet the nutritional needs of these exceedingly normal folks. Of course, if you weigh significantly more or less than those figures, you need to adjust accordingly. And similarly, if you're pregnant, lactating, postmenopausal, or a kid, your requirements are different from what the RDA suggests.

That said, here's something to keep in mind: a guideline for dietary intake is laid out in the USDA's Food Guide Pyramid, which breaks down the recommended number of servings for each of the five basic food groups. The groups are as follows:

◆ Bread, cereal, pasta, and rice
◆ Vegetables
◆ Fruit
◆ Milk, yogurt, and cheese
◆ Meat, poultry, fish, dry beans, eggs, and nuts

A sixth group, the one that makes most of us salivate, is pleasing to the palate but high in fat or calories. This group includes fats, oils, and sweets. Sadly, these substances have little (or no) nutritive value and should be eaten sparingly. (One can only imagine the frenzy caused by a study that said the best diet would include copious servings of ice cream, potato chips, mayonnaise, and bacon.)

Here's something else you should know: the six essential nutrients:

◆ Carbohydrates
◆ Proteins
◆ Fats
◆ Vitamins
◆ Minerals
◆ Water

Flex Facts

The Food Guide Pyramid provides a visual representation of a healthful diet, emphasizing the need for complex carbohydrates. And it's not some outdated information from the 1950s. The USDA updates the pyramid as warranted. Learn more at www.mypyramid.gov/.

Before we get into the nuts and bolts of what and when to eat, let's do a quickie course in basic nutrition.

Carbohydrates (carbs), proteins, and fats are your sources of calories. Carbs supply 4 calories per gram and are classified as simple or complex. This isn't a psychological profile, but it is based on the properties each possesses. Simple carbs, which are quickly converted to energy, are high in sugar and found in treats such as cakes, cookies, jams, and soda.

Complex carbohydrates, which provide a more sustained and gradual release of glucose into the bloodstream, are found in pasta, bread, grains, and cereals. Complex carbs should be the mainstay of your diet.

Fats don't provide a lot of vitamins and minerals, but they serve a valuable role in your diet. For example, without ingesting some fat—about 2 tablespoons a day—your body couldn't process or absorb vitamins A, D, E, or K.

Protein, which forms the structural basis for muscle tissue, supplies energy only when there aren't enough calories available from carbs and fat. Foods high in protein include meat, milk, eggs, and legumes.

That's the basics on what we eat. Many experts disagree on the precise figures, but it's our informed opinion that a good diet should consist of 60 to 65 percent carbohydrates, 10 to 12 percent protein, and 20 to 30 percent fat. Here's a helpful key to figure out how much of each type of food you should eat.

First you need to figure out your basal metabolic rate (BMR). Your BMR is the amount of energy (calories) you'd burn just to keep going if you did nothing but lie in bed staring at the wall. (The ultimate couch potato doesn't even use the remote control.) It's both amusing and informative to figure out the approximate number of calories your body needs each day to maintain your weight. To figure out your BMR for one day, get your calculator and punch in the following numbers. This estimate should be within 15 percent of your actual BMR.

Men: Body weight (pounds) × 24 ÷ 2.2

Women: Body weight (pounds) × 21 ÷ 2.2

For example: Jonathan weighs 172 pounds. To find out his metabolic rate, he multiplies 172 by 24, which is 4,128, which he divides by 2.2 to get 1,876. So without exercising, he needs to consume 1,876 calories each day to maintain his body weight, and thus, to lose weight, he needs to eat fewer than 1,876 calories. Now, Jonathan actually does more than lie prone for the day. In fact, he burns about 1,500 or so calories each day swimming, cycling, running, and lifting weights, which means he breaks even at more than 3,300 calories a day. (By way of comparison, the average sumo wrestler consumes 4,600 calories a day.) Being able to approximate your metabolic rate enables you to have an idea of how many calories your body needs each day.

Do You Need More?

As an aspiring body beautiful, you may be wondering if your caloric needs are different than the average. Should you eat some extra protein? Maybe less fat? Good questions.

The Truth About Protein

When it comes to strength training and building muscle, the role of protein is perhaps the most misunderstood. First, some facts: the RDA for protein is 0.8 grams per kilogram. For our prototypical 154-pound (70-kilogram) friend, that's 56 grams of protein a day, or about 1 cup (9 grams) milk, 2 eggs (12 grams), and a 4-ounce (32-gram) serving of chicken or beef. In other words, it's quite easy to meet the RDA requirement.

"Whoa, Nellie!" you may be saying. "You just said protein helps make up the actual structure of the muscle. If that's true, isn't it best to eat more protein?" At the risk of sounding like a politician on the campaign trail, the answer is "yes and no."

Although scientific evidence suggests that some strength and endurance athletes may benefit from protein intakes of as much as 1.5 to 2.0 times the RDA, this is probably not necessary or helpful for the vast majority of people. The catch-22 is that you're probably already downing well over the RDA and just don't know it. So before you start doing a Rocky Balboa on us and slurp raw-egg shakes before heading to the gym, know that recent studies show the average American consumes more than 100 grams of protein per day. So although you may need more than the RDA, you're likely already there.

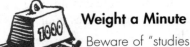

Weight a Minute

Beware of "studies" that claim you should consume more than twice the amount of protein suggested by the RDA. Odds are these are conducted by manufacturers of supplements who have a vested interest in your eating like a lion.

Water, Water, Everywhere

We cannot overstress the importance of proper hydration. Simply put, a human being can go for weeks without eating solid food but can't survive more than 3 to 7 days without water. A male's body is made up of 60 to 65 percent water; a female's, 50 to 60 percent. The human brain is about 75 percent water. Water aids in digestion and eases muscle soreness after a training session. Proper water consumption is crucial to weight loss.

Why, then, are most people, even serious athletes, underhydrated? The two most common answers we hear are: it's a nuisance, and maintaining proper hydration means you'll pee a lot. The first is debatable; the second is not.

In the course of a normal day—no naps in a sauna or foot races in the Gobi Desert—the average adult needs about 80 ounces of water to maintain water balance. Most people probably drink half that, which is why so many of us are sluggish, suffer from headaches, and feel stiff and sore after performing just a moderate amount of exercise.

If you exercise often (especially during the summer), drink a lot of coffee and booze (which act as diuretics), or take medication, you need to drink even more water. Even a slight drop in your body weight lost through perspiration can adversely affect your exercise performance. That means you should drink about 6 to 8 ounces of fluid every 15 minutes or so when you're exercising. On average, you should be consuming at least 8 ounces roughly 8 to 10 times a day.

Sound like a lot? Try it for a few days, and see how much better you feel.

Spot Me

During exercise, don't wait until you're thirsty to start drinking. By the time you're thirsty, you're well on your way to becoming dehydrated.

In short, making a lot of trips to the bathroom is a small price to pay when you consider how much better the human body functions when it's properly lubricated. Although water provides no energy (calories), your body can't use most of the nutrients it needs without water to process them.

Here are some salient facts about water:

- Water is responsible for providing the building materials for cell protoplasm. Don't ask, just trust us: it's important.
- Water helps protect the body's tissue and internal organs.
- Water helps regulate body temperature as well as transport other nutrients, hormones, and waste products.

There's more, but we assume you get the point by now: the more water you drink, the better you'll feel.

The Fancy Stuff

Okay, so water is cool, but what about Gatorade, Sportsade, and the scores of other liquid "ades" sprouting up all over the beverage aisle? After all, if it works for Michael Jordan, it's got to be good. Right? To which we reply unequivocally, "Maybe." Unless you're running, cycling, or engaging in any cardiovascular activity for at least 45 minutes to an hour a day or working out in a hot, humid gym, sports drinks really aren't necessary. Your body has no real physio-logical need for the extra calories or minerals in a sports drink. (You'll replenish everything you need in your next meal.)

> **Flex Facts** _____
> In the 1960s, a fluid replacement drink was developed at the University of Florida for the school's athletic teams, who train and play in hot, muggy weather nearly all year long. It's called Gatorade, named for the nickname of all the U of F teams—the Gators. Gatorade contains some vitamins and minerals, but it's mostly sugar and water.

However, if you are pounding the pavement with a vengeance, a sports drink may help you speed up the rate at which your body absorbs the fluid. Perhaps the biggest advantage these sporty drinks have over straight water is taste. A cold glass of pure mountain water may be the elixir of life, but after a while your taste buds may be calling out for more. Simply put, the more you like the taste, the more likely you are to drink the stuff.

Here are our top three tips for optimal hydration:

◆ Most commercial sports drinks contain a carbohydrate concentration of between 5 and 7 percent. Anything higher than that can cause gastric distress and actually slow fluid absorption. Diluted juice (50 percent juice/50 percent water) with maybe a pinch of salt works just as well.

◆ Drink 16 ounces of cold water or diluted sports drink before working out.

◆ Drink water every 15 minutes or so to prevent dehydration.

Lose It by the Book

We are a culture obsessed with weight, and for two reasons. First, we have before us the unre-alistic standards set by the incredibly thin super-models and actors who are viewed as "ideal." Second, we are the most overweight culture in the Western world. And oddly enough, despite our nation's keen interest in fitness, the obesity rates are on the rise.

If you're one of the millions of Americans struggling to lose weight, you're well aware of the countless products and diets promising to help you "drop those ugly pounds" in a matter of minutes. (Okay, days.) Not only are most of these products bogus, dangerous, or worse, even the best of them rarely produce long-term weight loss.

> **Spot Me** _____
> Try weighing yourself before and after a workout. If you're lighter after you train, it means you've lost more water from sweating than you've replenished in flu-ids. If that's the case, try drinking more next time. Remember, 1 pound of body weight is equivalent to 16 ounces of water.

Slow but Steady Wins the Race

With few exceptions, very low-calorie diets, skipping meals, and fasting are counterproduc-tive. When you make drastic adjustments to your caloric intake, your body's survival instincts sound an alarm and slow your metabolism to a snail's pace. Your goal is to speed up your metabolic rate, not the other way around. When you sit down to your next meal after a fast, your metabolism remains depressed, which actually causes you to gain weight.

Because most health experts agree that a weight loss of more than 2 pounds per week is unhealthy, we recommend a weekly goal of 1 pound. Usually, when you lose more than that per week, you're actually losing muscle as well as fat—a big no-no, because not only does muscle look good, but it also helps you burn calories.

To lose 1 pound a week, you need to burn 500 calories more than you ingest each day. That may seem like a formidable number, but it really isn't if you exercise. If you can manage to burn an extra 250 calories a day—a 2.5-mile jog or 30 minutes on the exercise bike—you're halfway there. Remember, your body won't know the difference if you get those miles walking to the post office in lieu of running in the park. Also keep in mind that as you increase your muscle mass, you'll be burning extra calories. Even as you read this book your muscles are metabolically active. (Reading this book while you walk to the post office is even better.)

Here are some handy ways to decrease the number of calories you eat each day:

◆ In the morning, eat a piece of whole-wheat toast instead of a bagel. *Calories saved:* 150.

◆ Hold the mayo and use mustard on your turkey sandwich. *Calories saved:* 100.

◆ Use tomato sauce (without sugar) instead of a creamy Alfredo on your pasta. *Calories saved:* 190.

◆ Use skim or low-fat soy milk in place of whole milk. *Calories saved:* 60.

◆ Pass on the midday candy bar snack and down a piece of fruit. *Calories saved:* 180. (If you're still hungry, eat raw nuts.)

◆ Toss that can of cola and drink water. *Calories saved:* 150.

◆ Use one instead of two sugars in your coffee. Better yet, use none. *Calories saved:* 15 to 30.

Flex Facts

Men with more than 25 percent body fat and women with more than 30 percent body fat are considered obese. Studies by the National Center of Health Statistics over the last two decades show that today approximately 35 percent of women and 31 percent of men age 20 and older are considered obese. That's an increase of approximately 30 percent and 25 percent, respectively, from 1980.

The Sad Truth About Fad Diets

As P. T. Barnum might have said, "A weight-loss sucker is born every minute." No matter how outrageous or absurd the alternative, many people refuse to apply common sense and sound science to their dietary needs (or their pocketbooks). Recently, we heard a radio spot for a product called "The Fat Assassin" that promised to melt off pounds quicker than you could spell John Wilkes Booth. Although the image is clearly preposterous, enough people are apparently buying it to justify the number of ads on the air.

You can learn the hard way or take our word for it right now: wacky diets such as the "Grapefruit Diet" or the "Cabbage Diet" that exclude or severely restrict whole categories of food do more harm than good because they typically exclude important vitamins and minerals.

Take Barry Sears's The Zone, a low-carbohydrate diet that in the 1990s gained more notoriety than Monica Lewinsky. A few years ago, one of the guys Jonathan trains with raved about how he'd lost 7 pounds in just a week by following Sears's 40-30-30 diet (40 percent of your daily calories from carbohydrates, 30 percent from protein, and 30 percent from fat). Basically, the premise of The Zone diet is that eating too many carbs makes you fat.

Jonathan, who seemingly gets joy from telling little children there's no Santa Claus, was more than happy to point out the flaw in The Zone theory. True, his training buddy had lost a whopping 7 pounds in 7 days; however, when you know that carbs, which are stored in the body as glycogen, hold three times their weight in water, you realize that this suddenly svelte Zone-ite had lost water and sugar, not fat. That's a good way to travel if you're like Deidre trying to make weight for a powerlifting competition, but useless if your aim is to drop fat. Once again, if something seems too good to be true, it probably is. In most cases, long-term weight loss from low-carbohydrate diets comes from the fact that the diets are also low in calories—not because they're low in carbs.

Flex Facts

Elite male marathoners generally carry about 4 to 6 percent body fat. Football linemen can range from 17 to 23 percent. When Deidre won her first World Powerlifting title, she carried 14 percent body fat. This triathlon season Jonathan is lugging 7 percent. Essential body fat, the amount necessary for normal physiologic function, is approximately 3 percent in men and 12 percent in women. These levels may interfere with normal function and are not necessary for optimal health. Males at 15 to 18 percent and females at 19 to 23 percent body fat are considered healthy.

A Pound of Feathers or a Pound of Rocks

As we've mentioned, the scale doesn't know the difference between 1 pound of water and 1 pound of fat. The same can be said about the difference between muscle and fat. Plainly put, "A pound is a pound is a pound" on the scale.

However, there's actually quite a huge difference between the way a pound of muscle and a pound of fat looks on the human body.

When clients tell Jonathan they're frustrated that they haven't lost weight despite their best efforts, he reminds them that they've dropped a dress size or a belt loop. The bottom line isn't what the scale says, but your ratio of fat to lean mass.

Take, for example, two chaps who stand 5 feet 10 inches and tip the scales at 180 pounds. Mr. Stud Muffin has only 10 percent (or 18 pounds) of body fat, while Mr. Potato Latke is schlepping 25 percent of his weight as fat. That means Mr. Latke has more than twice the fat of his counterpart. The scale can't tell them apart, but a measurement of their body fat sure can.

There are many ways to gauge your percentage of body fat—underwater weighing being the most accurate—but most knowledgeable trainers with skin-fold calipers can give you a reasonable assessment. However, the best way to see where you stand is to step in front of a mirror in the buff and look for yourself.

To Supplement or Not?

If you think eating right is a challenge, a trip through your local vitamin shop can be downright treacherous. Let's take a look at what supplements help you meet your fitness goals and which ones may not only fail to help and waste your money, but may actually harm you.

Buyer Beware

First of all, the most common dietary deficiencies are carbohydrates and fluids—neither of which require a trip to a health food store. Second, vitamin, protein, and mineral deficiency is rare in people with a balanced diet. You should also know that while a shortage of a nutrient can have a negative effect, taking an excess of one particular substance usually does more harm than good. For instance, a protein deficiency can leave you feeling sluggish, but ingesting excess protein can actually cause weight gain and kidney problems.

In 1989, the Food and Drug Administration (FDA) defined a dietary supplement as a substance made of essential nutrients such as vitamins, minerals, and *amino acids*. The following year, an act of legislation came down the pike broadening the term *dietary supplements* to include herbs and similar nutritional substances. Then in 1994, another act from the feds established yet another definition. Here are the rules that allow a company to identify and market a product as a dietary supplement today:

◆ The product must be labeled as a "dietary supplement."

◆ The product must contain one or more of the following ingredients: a vitamin, mineral, herb or other botanical, and amino acids. (There are other criteria, but they're too tedious to mention.)

◆ The product is intended for ingestion in pill, capsule, tablet, or liquid form. In other words, desiccated caterpillars from China fall outside the guidelines.

◆ The product must not be represented as a conventional food or as the sole item of a meal or diet. The Complete One-Pill Breakfast, Lunch, or Dinner ain't cuttin' it right now.

It's worth noting that these regulations require the manufacturer's statements to be "truthful and not misleading," but do not establish any standard for the often outrageous claims that supposedly back up such statements. In other words, a single study—even one financed by the manufacturer using shaky statistical methods— is enough, even if that one study contradicts scores of other more impartial studies. And you wonder how Jonathan became such a skeptic.

When you're browsing the aisles in your local health food store, study the fine print on the product's label. If you see "This statement has not been evaluated by the FDA," you should think *buyer beware*. Claims made on food labels are more strictly regulated than on supplement labels and hence must answer to a higher authority.

Before we get into some of the most popular individual supplements on the market, consider these random facts on dietary supplements:

◆ Supplements include vitamins and minerals, as well as herbals and botanicals.

◆ Multivitamins may help some people, but less is known about herbals and botanicals.

◆ High doses of certain supplements may be harmful.

◆ Don't assume *natural* means "safe." The two words are not synonymous. Tobacco is natural, and we know the often lethal long-term risks of using that product.

◆ If you want to ensure you're getting all you need, eat a variety of foods.

Powder Power

Earlier in this chapter, we discussed how most people get more than enough protein in their diet. However, occasionally vegetarians or folks on low-calorie diets may be protein-deficient. Even if you fall into that category, there's no reason to run out and buy a tub of Super Mega Muscle Man Protein Powder you may have seen advertised in a fitness magazine.

In grad school, Jonathan had occasion to examine such a powder. The label of this "miracle" mix of muscle-building powder purported to have the ideal combination of amino acids, which are the building blocks of protein. According to the directions, the optimal way to use the powder was to mix it with a glass of skim milk. However, on closer inspection,

Jonathan and his classmates determined that at least one third of the amino acids in this miraculous concoction came from the skim milk. Considering that the powder cost a few bucks per serving and the milk retailed for roughly 20¢, all you had to do was down three glasses of skim milk, and you'd have achieved the same effect. If you're totally sold on powders, try evaporated nonfat dry milk. Anti-dairy? Soy milk or rice milk should fit the bill.

Weight a Minute

Don't believe everything you read. Many of the manufacturers of the supplements advertised in some of the most popular "muscle" and fitness magazines own the magazine their products appear in. If that's the case, don't expect an unbiased opinion of a product.

The Creatine Craze

Talk to serious weight lifters, cyclists, swimmers, and a host of athletes from a cross-section of sports, and odds are they've tried creatine. What is it? And why take it?

Creatine, a nitrogen-containing compound naturally found in our bodies, is made by the liver, kidneys, and pancreas. Creatine helps provide the energy your muscles need to move, particularly when they make movements that require short bursts of explosive energy such as that required in weight lifting.

When your muscles contract, the fuel that initiates this movement is a catchy-sounding compound called adenosine triphosphate (ATP). There's only enough ATP in your body to provide energy for roughly 10 seconds, meaning that for this energy system to continue functioning, the body must produce more ATP. We'll spare you the chemistry lesson, but trust us that creatine acts like an oxygen tank to a

high-altitude mountaineer, assisting the body to produce more ATP, which in turn can be used as fuel for more muscle contraction. Because the ability to regenerate ATP depends on one's supply of creatine, it appears that upping creatine levels in your muscles allows for greater ATP resynthesis. If, in fact, all the above is true, ATP resynthesis prevents your body from relying on your other energy systems, which are not as powerful when relied upon to produce explosive movements.

Does creatine work? Probably—especially for vegetarians, because creatine is found in most meats and fish. However, no matter how much sushi or creatine you ingest, the mere fact that you take creatine won't make you stronger. It's only effective if you work harder in the gym.

Is it safe? Good question. In the short term, it appears to produce no serious side effects, but it's hard to say over the long haul because studies have yet to be done to measure its effects over time. Some folks who use it complain about gastrointestinal discomfort or muscle cramps, which is probably due to a lack of fluid intake. Proper hydration should alleviate the problem. In powder form, taking creatine is a bit like eating dishwashing detergent. It comes in pills as well, which are far easier to swallow but may not be absorbed as effectively. Weight gain often accompanies creatine use because you're likely to retain a little extra water in the muscle as well as experience muscle growth.

One last tip: most creatine manufacturers recommend a "loading" phase of 20 grams a day for the first week or more, followed by a more moderate "maintenance" dose of 2 to 5 grams a day. There has been very little proof that this loading phase actually increases your creatine stores rather than just causing the excess to be excreted by the liver and kidneys. We suggest that you experiment. Go right to the maintenance phase, and see if you feel a difference. If so, we've saved you a few bucks.

(Creatine is nearly $30 a bottle for 120 gel capsules or 500 grams of powder.)

DHEA, Andro, Chromium, Ephedrine

Today's hot new magic pill often turns out to be tomorrow's debunked placebo or dangerous, outlawed garbage. Once upon a time, DHEA, androstendione, chromium picolinate, ephedrine, and guarana were touted as the next big advancement in ergogenic aids.

Today, andro (androstendione) and DHEA (dehydroepiandrosterone) are outlawed by the International Olympic Committee, the NCAA, Major League Baseball, and the National Football League. Although they may possess some legitimate benefits—especially for the elderly—no legitimate research yet supports their use in healthy young or middle-aged adults. On the other hand, ample evidence shows taking andro can lead to increased breast size in men, and some studies suggest these hormones can increase the risk of certain cancers and in reducing testicular size in men.

Ephedrine was a popular metabolic booster purported to help promote weight loss. Unfortunately, it's a central nervous system stimulant that can have dangerous side effects and has been implicated in numerous deaths, including those of Baltimore Orioles pitcher Steve Belcher in 2002 and Minnesota Vikings offensive lineman Korey Stringer in 2001. Today, ephedrine is illegal, but for years it was used by recreational and elite athletes as well as sedentary dieters. It's a good reminder that just because something is legal and available at your local supplement store doesn't mean that it's safe or effective.

Burn, Baby, Burn

A few years back, another supposed wonder substance was chromium picolinate—a supplement that, according to its advocates, can do anything from help you lose weight to gain muscle mass to speed your metabolism. Scientific evidence, however, suggests otherwise.

Chromium's role in the body is to help tissues respond efficiently to insulin, which helps keep blood sugar levels in balance. However, although the natural substance plays an essential physiological role in the body, it's highly questionable whether its supplementation has any *ergogenic* effect on people with normal insulin or blood sugar levels. In other words, you can't live without the stuff, but it's unlikely that taking it in supplement form does much more than improve your ability to swallow pills.

Bar Talk

An **ergogenic** aid is any product that improves athletic or physical performance.

Starbucks, Anyone?

In the "old" days, you could get a good cup of coffee in New York City for 50¢. Today, in the era of gourmet coffee shops, half a buck gets you into the men's room. Simply put, coffee has become big business. While you can drop $3.50 for a mocha latte cappuccino at Starbucks, caffeine—a substance banned by the International Olympic Committee—is one of the cheapest and perhaps most beneficial ergogenic aids out there. (Just for the record: to get booted from the Olympics for abusing caffeine you'd have to top out way above the dose that is allowable and most beneficial.)

Caffeine works to help you in two ways. During aerobic activities, it can increase the availability of fat as fuel. And although it won't make you stronger during weight lifting, some evidence shows that caffeine helps make the activity *seem* easier.

Before you start swilling shots of espresso, keep the following in mind:

- ◆ Caffeine can cause gastrointestinal problems.
- ◆ Drinking too much can make you jittery.
- ◆ Caffeine is a diuretic. Drink extra water if you're going to work up a sweat.
- ◆ Possible links exist between caffeine consumption and benign fibrocystic breast disease.
- ◆ If you have an ulcer or irregular heartbeat, your best bet is to stick to decaf.

Weight a Minute

HMB (hydroxymethylbutyrate), pyruvate, inosine, branch-chained amino acids, bee pollen, and ginseng are other rather popular supplements you've probably heard about. None of them impress us for a variety of reasons, mainly because we're concerned about whether they're safe and effective.

The Bar Scene

Flip through any bicycle or runner's apparel catalogue and you're bound to see a host of ads for energy bars such as PowerBar, Clif Bar,

Met-Rx Bar, Balance Bar, PR Ironman Bar, and the list goes on. Each makes bold claims about what it can do for you, from optimizing your body's natural ability to burn stored fat for energy to providing you with a burst of energy. Not only are they supposed to start your engine and keep it running at optimal efficiency, they're designed to taste good (unlike their ancestors, which tasted a tad better than the rubber flooring in your gym). Check out some of these flavors: white chocolate mocha, berry blast, cookie dough, and Kona crunch. Sounds like a get-together at a Ben & Jerry's convention.

These smartly marketed products are good under a variety of conditions, including when you're doing a long training ride, are too hungry to work out but too busy to eat, and as a late-night snack when a piece of fruit just doesn't have enough *oomph*. Most of these bars are easily digested and pack a fair number of nutrients in a convenient package. When Jonathan wakes up at the obscene hour of 5 A.M. for a bike race, he's usually too comatose to prepare breakfast and simply downs a PowerBar as a pre-race meal.

Here are a few energy bar tidbits:

- ◆ Most bars are fairly high in carbohydrates, which are more readily digested than calories from protein or fat.
- ◆ Some, however, are extremely high in protein and may not be easy to digest. As we've said, extra protein often does more harm than good.
- ◆ Beware of bars that make outrageous claims. These bars are a good source of food to help stabilize blood sugar levels and fight hunger pangs, but they're not

going to make you burn fat faster. And they're not going to make you stronger or faster. Despite what he and the advertisers may say, six-time Ironman Triathlon winner Mark Allen didn't run down his competition because he ate PR Bars. (In fact, given his talent and training regimen, he could have eaten a bar of soap and still dominated.)

From A to Zinc

One of the most interesting facts about vitamin and mineral supplementation is that more often than not, if you believe taking them is good for you, it is. In other words, the power of the mind to invest positive qualities in things we believe are good for us is not to be denied. (Studies on the placebo effect are nothing short of remarkable: patients with inoperative cancer who were given a "miracle" cure [sugar pills] actually saw their cancer temporarily go into remission.)

That said, both competitive and recreational athletes tend to overdose on vitamins and minerals, considering that most people who eat a balanced diet get more than enough from the foods they eat. However, the most common vitamins missing in our diets are B_6, B_{12} (typically found in animal products), E (found in vegetable oils), and folic acid (found in leafy green vegetables and organ meats). In addition, many women don't get enough calcium and iron in their diet.

Megadosing on vitamins is probably a waste of time and money—and in the case of fat-soluble vitamins and minerals, detrimental—but taking a multivitamin can serve as a safe, inexpensive insurance policy against deficiencies caused by poor diet.

The Least You Need to Know

◆ Sound nutrition starts with sound science.

◆ When it comes to building muscle, protein is the most misunderstood food group.

◆ Proper hydration is crucial, but sports drinks have their place in the diets of serious athletes.

◆ Eschew fad diets and practice the only real way to lose weight: moderation, variety, and balance.

◆ The scale doesn't lie, but it doesn't tell the whole truth. Your percentage of body fat is just as important as how much you weigh.

◆ Nutritional supplements are big business. Read the labels and beware of outrageous claims.

In This Chapter

- ◆ Understanding the importance of a medical checkup
- ◆ Heeding medical precautions and prescriptions
- ◆ Handling injuries
- ◆ Learning the medical benefits of weight training
- ◆ Practicing safety
- ◆ Making your way around the gym
- ◆ Playing nice: courtesy counts in the gym

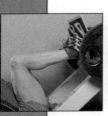 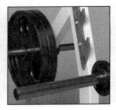 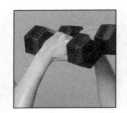 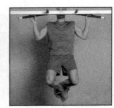 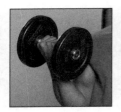 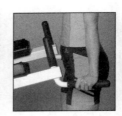

3

Getting a Clean Bill of Health

Here's an amusing paradox: when you're sick or injured, it's nearly impossible to think or talk about anything other than your health or lack of it. When Joe broke his wrist before his kayaking season a while back, he had to muzzle himself not to mention it to perfect strangers. "Excuse me, sir, I've broken one of my carpal bones. Care to hear this gripping tale?" Conversely, there's almost nothing more tedious on Earth than listening to someone tell you about his health problems. Unless, of course, you have the same condition. In fact, put three guys with broken wrists in a room together, provide refreshments, and they'll entertain themselves till the bones heal.

We note this phenomenon because of the importance of consulting with your physician before taking to the gym, and knowing what you need to be aware of—medically speaking—when you embark on a new exercise regimen. Given its clinical nature, this section may seem a bit on the dry side. On the other hand, we offer you some important information about how to keep yourself healthy and strong while working out to get even healthier and stronger. If it's been a while since you've had a checkup or exercised on a regular basis, or if you've had (or have) a serious medical condition, you need to take special care. But there's good news: very few people need to be excluded from working out—although modifications may be necessary. Read on for more info.

The Medical Checkup

The prudent path to follow when you're starting a weight-lifting regimen is to see your doctor for a thorough checkup. Again, this is especially important if you've been inactive for a while, have a bad back, are overweight, or are over 45. To some, getting a checkup is an odious task. Assuming your doctor is a decent sort, it shouldn't be. In health and fitness (as in virtually anything else), knowledge is power. Think of getting a physical not as a burden but as an opportunity to become more powerful.

Okay, let's say you haven't been sick in 10 years, you're 29 years old, and the idea of visiting a doctor is as appealing as having a root canal. The generally accepted minimal standard to gauge if you're ready to work out is a seven-question self-evaluation called the Physical Activity Readiness Questionnaire (PAR-Q). Designed for people between the ages of 15 and 69, it was developed by the Canadian Society for Exercise Physiology to see if you've got the mettle to push some metal.

PAR-Q and YOU
(A Questionnaire for People Aged 15 to 69)

Regular physical activity is fun and healthy, and more people are starting to become increasingly active every day. Being more active is very safe for most people. However, some people should check with their doctor before they start becoming physically active.

If you are planning to become much more physically active than you are now, start by answering the seven questions below. If you are between the ages of 15 and 69, the PAR-Q will tell you if you should check with your doctor before you start. If you are over 69 years of age, and you are not used to being very active, check with your doctor.

Common sense is your best guide when you answer these questions. Please read the questions carefully and answer each one honestly: check YES or NO.

Yes	No	
❏	❏	1. Has your doctor ever said that you have a heart condition and that you should only do physical activity recommended by a doctor?
❏	❏	2. Do you feel pain in your chest when you do physical activity?
❏	❏	3. In the past month, have you had chest pain when you were not doing physical activity?
❏	❏	4. Do you lose your balance because of dizziness, or do you ever lose consciousness?
❏	❏	5. Do you have a bone or joint problem that could be made worse by a change in your physical activity?
❏	❏	6. Is your doctor currently prescribing drugs (for example, water pills) for your blood pressure or heart condition?
❏	❏	7. Do you know of any other reason why you should not do physical activity?

If you answered …

YES to one or more questions

Talk with your doctor by phone or in person BEFORE you start to become much more physically active or before you have a fitness appraisal. Tell your doctor about the PAR-Q and which questions you answered YES.

- You may be able to do any activity you want—as long as you start slowly and build up gradually. Or, you may need to restrict your activities to those which are safe for you. Talk with your doctor about the kinds of activities you wish to participate in and follow his/her advice.
- Find out which community programs are safe and helpful for you.

NO to all questions

If you answered NO to *all* PAR-Q questions, you can be reasonably sure that you can:

- Start becoming much more physically active—begin slowly and build up gradually. This is the safest and easiest way to go.
- Take part in a fitness appraisal—this is an excellent way to determine your basic fitness so that you can plan the best way for you to live actively.

DELAY BECOMING MUCH MORE ACTIVE …

- If you are not feeling well because of a temporary illness such as a cold or a fever—wait until you feel better; or
- If you are or may be pregnant—talk to your doctor before you start becoming more active.

  Please note: if your health changes so that you then answer YES to any of the above questions, tell your fitness or health professional. Ask whether you should change your physical activity plan.

Informed use of the PAR-Q: The Canadian Society for Exercise Physiology, Health Canada, and their agents assume no liability for persons who undertake physical activity, and if in doubt after completing this questionnaire, consult your doctor prior to physical activity.

If you answer yes to any of these questions, or if you're older than 69, head straight to your doctor's office and tell the doctor you responded in the affirmative to one of the questions on the Physical Activity Readiness Questionnaire. Then let him or her give you a good once-over.

On the other hand, if you honestly answered no to these probing questions, the PAR-Q says it's okay to go ahead and have at it—but only if you do so gradually and follow all the safety precautions we outline for you throughout the book. (Just to put our prudent approach in perspective: even if you're in tremendous physical condition, it's unwise to start a new regimen like a lifter possessed. Starting out too fast is a sure way to get injured, even if you're fit.)

Most people over the age of 50 or so are concerned about heart disease, and for good reason. Heart attacks and strokes remain the single biggest killers in the United States. Because exercising puts extra strain on your heart and blood vessels, you need to be especially careful to be sure your cardiovascular system is in good working order. Here are the risk factors for coronary artery disease set forth by the American College of Sports Medicine. See where you stack up under any of the following categories:

- **Age.** Men over the age of 45; women over 55, or who have premature menopause without estrogen replacement therapy.

- **A family history of heart attacks or strokes.** Or sudden death of your father (or another close male relative) before the age of 55. Ditto for your mother (or close female relative) before the age of 65. Genes are powerful, so don't stick your head in the sand if your family's history is sketchy. Go get checked out.

- **Cigarette smoking.** Anyone who can read knows smoking contributes to lung cancer, heart disease, and a host of other physical problems. We'll spare you the lecture, but if you smoke and want to work out, see your doctor before you launch a fitness regimen. Of course, it's better to work out and smoke than to just smoke, but our guess is that the more you get into the gym, the less you'll suck the cigarettes.

- **Hypertension.** Exercise is one of the best antidotes for this condition, often curing the condition without the need for medication, but you'll need to be sure you're not stressing an already stressed-out circulatory system. See your doc if you've got any doubts.

- **High cholesterol.** Volumes have been written about good and bad cholesterol— what's high, what's low, what's dangerous, and what's not. Your doctor can tell you what's best for you, but a good rule of thumb is if your total cholesterol is more than 200 mg/dl or if your HDL or "good cholesterol" is below 35 mg/dl, you are considered at risk. (For the record, mg/dl means milligrams per deciliter.) Again, exercise will have a beneficial effect in increasing your HDL, but be sure you're not an egg yolk away from doing yourself serious harm.

- **Diabetes mellitus.** The connection between diabetes and heart disease is well known, so if you've been insulin-dependent for more than 15 years or are over age 30 with diabetes, you're considered at risk. The same is true of those non–insulin-dependent diabetics over 35.

- **Physical inactivity.** If your job keeps you pasted to your seat most of the day, or if the most arduous thing you've done in a year or more is play badminton at the company picnic, you're considered at risk if you engage in strenuous physical activity.

These risk factors don't mean you shouldn't or can't work out, but you should exercise a little extra caution before you get started. And the first step you take should be to the doctor's office.

A "normal" healthy blood pressure is around 120/80. Hypertension, or high blood pressure, is defined as any reading of 140/90 or more. By definition, blood pressure is the pressure exerted on the wall of a blood vessel. The first number, or systolic pressure, occurs as the heart contracts, while the second, diastolic pressure, occurs when the heart relaxes between beats.

"The Doctor Will See You Now"

Weight training can help treat a variety of ailments, especially if it's combined with a good stretching program and sound nutrition. We're not going to be so bold as to say that weight training can cure serious maladies like beriberi or foot-and-mouth disease, but it often does wonders for an ailing body. Having said that, weight lifting will exacerbate a number of conditions if you lift without medical supervision.

We don't mean to dampen your enthusiasm or frighten you off the exercise train; in fact, that's the last thing we want to do—well, the second to the last. We're most eager to help you avoid injuries or aggravate a preexisting condition. It may seem obvious, but we'll mention it anyway: when you're having a checkup, be sure to mention any current problems you're experiencing. In other words, don't try to turn the doctor into a mind reader. Once you've had your physical and learned how to safely proceed, find out if the gym you belong to (or are thinking about joining) has trainers who know how to work around your particular condition. Working with a trainer who isn't adept at working with stroke victims or heart patients—if that's your problem—is a big mistake.

Avoiding Risky Business

Okay, so you have high blood pressure or some other medical condition that provides a convenient excuse not to work out. Know this: $\frac{9}{10}$ tenths of the physical restrictions people live with are self-imposed. A few years back, a man with AIDS ran, cycled, and swam across the United States to prove to himself (and others) that people with this life-threatening disease can do far more than anyone realized. Just to drive home the point further: a man paralyzed from the waist down climbed Yosemite's El Capitan, one of the grandest rock faces in the world. At Joe and Deidre's gym, a woman with an artificial right arm lifts weights.

Let's look at some of the more common afflictions people have to deal with as they pertain to working out.

Hyper Types

Hypertension, or high blood pressure, is a condition that affects millions of Americans by placing chronic, increased stress on the normal function of the cardiovascular system. Often called the silent killer, hypertension is particularly insidious because it often goes undetected until you see the doctor or even have a heart attack or stroke.

Deidre has a photo taken of her deadlifting 365 pounds during a powerlifting competition. What's striking about it, besides the fact that she's lifting the equivalent of a baby elephant, is the terrific strain that shows on her face: her eyes bulge like Marty Feldman's and the veins in her neck are engorged like bloated worms. (We call this the Beauty and the Beast syndrome.) Few of us are likely to try to hoist that amount of weight, but the fact remains that weight lifting can increase your blood pressure during the actual exercise.

A common mistake is holding your breath during a repetition. We talk more about this once we get you into the gym, but for now, it's worth mentioning that holding your breath is ill advised—with high blood pressure or without. Competitive lifters like Deidre often hold their breath when they're shooting for a personal record (PR), but doing so may cause you bodily harm.

Weight a Minute

Holding your breath while lifting causes an exaggerated and sometimes dangerously high increase in blood pressure. The technical term for holding your breath during a lift is a *Valsalva maneuver*.

Post-Stroke Fitness

For some stroke victims, embarking on a weight-lifting program can be an essential part of their recovery. For others, doing so can be downright dangerous. If you have had a stroke, you need to discuss weight training with your doctor to see which category of patient you fall in.

Typically, if one side of your body is impaired or severely restricted, a knowledgeable physical therapist or trainer will have you work a lot on your unaffected side, because this part of your body will now be working much harder to compensate.

Deidre, who has worked for years as a physical therapist, has done a lot of work with stroke victims and is continually amazed by the progress people are able to make. One of her most remarkable patients is a woman in her 80s who had a stroke 12 years ago. She was unable to use her right arm and was able to walk with the use of a brace on her right leg and a cane. She walked outside, alone, every day and was able to cook and clean for herself.

Post–Heart-Attack Workout

For some, a heart attack spells the beginning of the end. Victims sense their own mortality and just "try and take it easy," which does little except make them sluggish and more prone to poor health. For others, surviving heart disease is like a second lease on life and a chance to nurture health instead of abuse it or take it for granted.

If you've had a heart attack or are at high risk for one, your doctor may well suggest you join a cardiac rehabilitation program—which has strict guidelines for cardiovascular as well as strength-training exercise—or simply encourage you to start exercising slowly. In the latter case, it's wise to work with a trainer or physical therapist who specializes in cardiac rehab. Combining aerobic activity, which can strengthen your heart (which is, after all, a muscle), and a sound diet will no doubt change your life.

Breathing Right

Asthma is a nasty affliction with symptoms that include wheezing, chest congestion, chest tightness, coughing, or shortness of breath. Exercising in cold, dry air is usually the most troublesome for asthmatics, while activities such as swimming are often tolerated much better. Usually, a thorough warm-up before exercise can help prevent symptoms, and many athletes with asthma have risen to the top of their game. Just look at former marathon world record–holder Alberto Salazar or Olympic gold medalist Jackie Joyner-Kersee, both diagnosed with asthma. Jonathan also has asthma, but nevertheless may be the best athlete in his apartment building. (Actually, Jonathan, who was severely afflicted with asthma as a child, has benefited greatly from exercise, and though he never trains without his inhaler, his condition no longer prevents him from competing.)

Flex Facts _____

During the 1992 Summer Olympics, many television viewers were shocked to find out that track and field champion Jackie Joyner-Kersee suffered from asthma. Joyner-Kersee is perhaps the greatest woman athlete ever, and her performance proved that asthma does not prevent exercise, even given the demands of top-level competition.

Today, with the advances in medications that can help prevent or alleviate symptoms with few side effects, asthmatics have every reason to exercise if they choose. Your doctor can prescribe an inhaler, which you should keep with you whenever you're exercising in case symptoms arise.

The Sugar Blues

Diabetes is a disease in which an insufficient amount of insulin (a hormone necessary for the metabolism of blood glucose or blood sugar) is produced by the body. This leads to an abnormally high blood glucose level. When the body functions normally, it releases insulin to counteract the increased sugar as blood glucose levels rise after eating. In diabetics, the body does not release enough insulin (as in the case of Type I, juvenile onset diabetes), or the body is insulin resistant, in which case insulin doesn't do what it's supposed to (as in the more common, Type II, adult onset diabetes). If the blood sugar level dips, extreme hunger pangs and dizziness result. If it's bad enough, blackouts and/or diabetic shock follow.

Because some exercise can have an "insulin-like" effect, sometimes insulin dosages need to be altered after you begin an exercise program. Furthermore, where you inject the insulin may have to be changed because injecting into a working muscle may increase the rate the insulin is absorbed.

Adult onset diabetes can be cured or drastically improved by changes in your diet. If you do regulate your diabetes this way, be sure you eat before working out. Talk to your doctor or a nutritionist about the best time to structure your workouts so they coincide with your normal blood sugar levels.

Building Bones

Years ago it was considered "unladylike" for women to lift weights. Now medical science has come around to tell us that taking to the gym is an effective way for postmenopausal women to combat osteoporosis, a disease that causes the loss of bone density. A proper diet that includes plenty of calcium and magnesium and a gradual weight-training program can work wonders to prevent the disease from developing. Once osteoporosis has set in, however, it's important for you to get clearance from your doctor to determine if it's safe to lift weights.

Bum Knees

There seems to be an endless number of things that can cause your knees to ache—from running to poor posture to ballroom dancing. Sometimes postural awareness can cure your knees, sometimes a stretching program will alleviate your pain. If you pursue those remedies and your knees still ache, have your doctor check them out. Once you get the go-ahead, go easy. Very often, strengthening the muscles in your quadriceps and hamstrings will ease your pain.

Oy, My Back

Back pain is one of the most complicated issues in the medical profession. Your back is made of literally hundreds of bones, muscles, ligaments, and nerves—any of which can go on the fritz, depending on what you're doing and the amount of stress you're under. Consult a doctor if you're experiencing serious trouble. Some people have good results with chiropractors; others respond to massage and/or yoga. A book that has helped thousands of back-pain sufferers is *Healing Back Pain* (Warner Books, 1991) by Dr. John Sarno.

The basis of Sarno's premise is that anxiety and repressed anger trigger muscle spasm. While the pain is real and often debilitating, the onset is mental. Some people consider Sarno full of helium; others swear by him. Our advice is, if you suffer from chronic back pain your doctor can't seem to "fix," hobble down to your bookstore and read what Sarno has to say.

Atlas Shrugged

The shoulder is an amazing joint. Maybe the credit belongs to our simian ancestors, who swung through the trees with the greatest of ease, but the range of motion the shoulder provides the arm is just short of miraculous. Think of a swimmer doing windmills to warm up for a race, or the last time you threw a Hail Mary pass in a touch football game.

But it's because the shoulder is so mobile and flexible that it's also so prone to injury. Shoulder injuries are one of the most common maladies caused by weight lifting—generally from lifting too much weight with too little form. Weight lifting can also aggravate an existing minor injury.

The two "itises"—*tendonitis* and *bursitis*—as well as *rotator cuff* tears, are all common injuries brought on by repetitive activity, such as racket sports and swimming. They all result in the same symptom: shoulder pain. It's normal for your shoulders to feel sore after serious exertion, like helping your cousin Ruth move to a fourth-floor walk-up or playing a game of ultimate Frisbee. But if it's been business as usual and you experience shoulder pain at rest or on movement, see your doctor.

Bar Talk

Anything that ends in "itis" means inflammation. **Tendonitis** is an inflammation of the tendons (the connective tissue that connects bone to muscle), and **bursitis** is an inflammation of the bursa (pad-like sacs found between tendons and bones that act to reduce friction).

One last bit of advice on a question that comes up far too often about the merits of working out when you're feeling under the weather. Ready for this political answer? Sometimes it can help, and sometimes it can hurt. Generally speaking, if all you have is a cold, and all your symptoms are above your neck (sniffles, tickly throat, etc.), a moderate workout can help clear your head. If your symptoms have spread to your chest or include fever or body aches, working out is likely to worsen the condition, so we suggest you rest, recover, and have at it when you're feeling better.

Safety in the Gym

Just because you've gotten the all-clear from your doctor doesn't mean you're free of danger. In fact, the gym can be a very treacherous place. After finishing several sets on the bench press years ago, Joe and a friend were removing 45-pound plates from either side of the barbell. Protocol dictates that each person remove the plates more or less at the same time. Joe, however, wasn't paying attention and removed all the weight from his end before his friend grabbed his side. The weighted side made like a seesaw, and the plate fell smack on his friend's big toe. Later on they had a good laugh about "Crack-a-toe-a," but at the time, Joe's momentary lapse left his friend hobbled for weeks.

Understanding safety issues in the gym is extremely important. People do get injured in health clubs, and more often than not the injury could have been avoided. Jonathan has lost count of the number of times he's had to sprint from one end of the gym to the other to pull a bar off the chest of a beefy dude who thought a spotter was reserved for the scrawny types.

There aren't a lot of gym safety rules, and they're not terribly complicated, but they are specific to this unique environment where motivated individuals (many of whom are wearing headphones) are hoisting large metal objects overhead.

Let's take a look at proper gym etiquette, correct form, and common safety concerns such as being sure the barbell collars are in place, being mindful where you drop your weights, and the right way to "spot" for someone. The key is consideration and awareness. If you were only in danger of hurting yourself, that would be one thing, but you become a threat to others if you start turning toes into pancakes on a regular basis.

Form, Form (and Form)

Hang out in a gym long enough, and you hear a litany of complaints—injured shoulders, stiff backs, tweaked biceps, and strained hamstrings. The causes are many and varied, but the biggest culprit is bad technique. Proper technique is the key not only to making solid strength gains, but also to maintaining health over the long term.

Generally speaking, using good form means lifting *less* weight than you might think you're able. Proper form requires you to isolate the muscle or muscles you're trying to build, which makes the exercise harder to perform.

We give you a complete description of the proper way to execute each exercise we recommend in the appropriate chapters, but you should keep in mind that the actual amount of weight you lift is in many ways insignificant.

Instead, what's important is how you lift that weight. Remember that you're lifting to improve your body and mind, not to pump up your ego. Lifting slowly through a full range of motion is your ultimate goal. If you practice proper technique from the beginning, you'll build a solid base—strength from the inside out. Slow, controlled movements and proper breathing are a few of the key components we stress.

Spot Me

By practicing proper form, you maximize the benefits of lifting while minimizing the danger. Never try to squeeze out an extra rep at the expense of form or safety.

What Goes Where?

The first time you walk into a gym you might feel like a city slicker dropped off in the middle of a forest. The texture of the landscape is so foreign you might feel dizzy with anxiety and confusion. But don't feel bad: to the uninitiated, the gym is a jungle, and you don't know where anything goes or what any of these shiny metal contraptions do.

Fret not! Once you learn the lay of the land, you'll waltz through the establishment like a deer bounding through the woods. In the following section, we discuss the typical layout of most gyms, where you'll find what, and what you should do with it once you're done using it. Here's a theoretical tour of a typical gym.

The Machines

Most gyms are set up just like a supermarket—all the equipment that's used for a particular body part is together just the way all the dairy products are in one aisle. Generally, machines are grouped so the machines that work larger muscles like chest and back come first, followed by those that work the smaller muscles like biceps and triceps. (As we explain later, that's the logical progression for you to follow in your routine.)

Sometimes, larger gyms have full lines of more than one brand of machines. If that's the case, you may find all the machines of one line grouped together and the other company's machines in another area. The point is that most gyms have a logical plan that's easy to discern once you know what to look for.

The Freeweights

The dumbbell racks are usually set up in front of a mirror according to weight, with the lighter weights on the top tier—say 5- to 50-pound dumbbells—and the heavier weights on the bottom tier. (The heaviest dumbbells we've seen in a gym are 150 pounders, which work well as anchors for ocean liners but which you shouldn't even consider trying to lift for some time.)

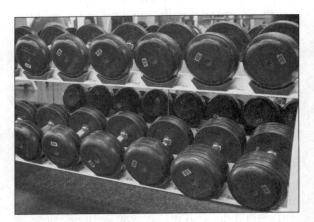

Dumbbell racks in tiers.

There are also odd-looking treelike objects (vertical racks) usually set up adjacent to the location of a barbell. These racks hold metal *plates* and are (we hope) arranged so the plates that weigh the same amount are grouped together. These plates can be as light as 2½ pounds and as heavy as 45 pounds. Unfortunately, when you're short on time, the 5-pound plate you really want invariably is buried under six

45-pounders—getting that out is a task nearly as arduous as digging out from under a train wreck!

Bar Talk

Plates are what you add to each side of a bar to increase its weight. Plates you'll see in most gyms come in denominations of 2½, 5, 10, 25, 35, and 45 pounds.

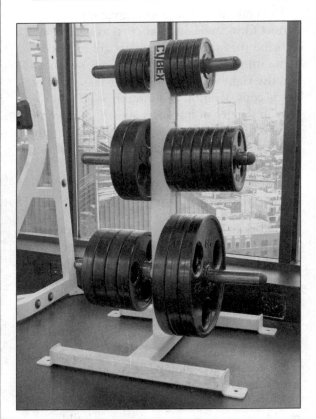

Plates on a tree.

The Bars

The long, 45-pound bar used in almost all commercial gyms is called an Olympic bar. These hefty rods of steel are usually found either on the various benches and racks or propped up in a corner. By adding plates to the bar and securing them with collars, you can control the amount of weight you lift for any given exercise. Some folks may use the bar alone when they bench press; others load as much as 500 pounds onto it. Assuming you're not working out with someone significantly stronger or weaker than you are (requiring you to remove and replace hundreds of pounds of weight), changing the weight is relatively easy. You just remove the collars, add or subtract weight, and continue on.

For those who aren't ready for a 45-pound bar on a particular exercise, lighter, shorter versions of the Olympic bar are usually available. They are the same diameter and just as compatible with the same set of plates.

Some of the larger and better-equipped gyms have "fixed" barbells in addition to Olympic bars. These bars are already loaded with plates in 5-pound increments and save you the time and trouble of loading and unloading the bar. These usually come in increments from 20 pounds up through 100 pounds. Beyond that, you're back to the bare Olympic bars.

The Pins

Unlike freeweights, which are as basic as a hammer and anvil, weight machines have more variables to concern yourself with. In fact, you're bound to encounter machines from lots of companies (Cybex, Nautilus, Bodymaster, Paramount, Maxicam, and more). Luckily, they are more alike than they are different.

Almost all of them are adjusted with pins. Pins are metal rods used to adjust a stack of weights on a particular machine. By placing the pin into a notch on the stack, you set how much weight you'll attempt to lift. Some pins fit straight into the weight stack, while others need to be inserted at a certain angle. Other machines require that you push a button before removing or inserting the pin.

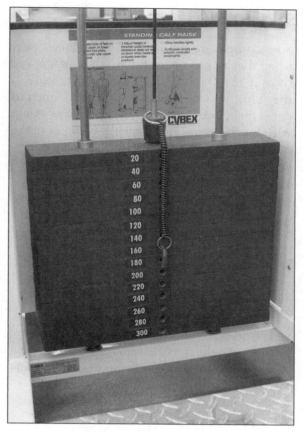

Weight stack using a pin.

Much like socks in a dryer, pins often disappear mysteriously. (Where they go, no one seems to know; because they have virtually no other use, theft is not a viable explanation.) If you're unable to find a pin for the machine you're using, contact a staff member.

One important note: never take a pin from one machine to use with another unless it's of the same model. Because the size and configuration of machines and their weight stacks vary, using the pin from a Universal machine on a Nautilus machine is ill advised. Often the pin will pop out and you'll be in for a rude surprise.

Ask First, Lift Later

Some people are comfortable asking questions when they're lost or confused, while others (usually men!) remain silent, even if it means they must wander aimlessly for hours. Much to our surprise, we consistently see people working out who clearly are clueless when it comes to the nuances of a particular machine. "Nuances my ear," you say. "This is a gym, not an art gallery!" Well, okay, let's just say that just about every piece of equipment can be adjusted in a variety of ways. For example, many benches can be set to a different angle, certain machines can be adjusted to your specifications, and some bars are better suited for certain exercises than others. It can be confusing until you learn which end is up.

Just as you wouldn't wander aimlessly around your workplace during the first week on the job, you shouldn't work out at the gym trying to figure out each piece of equipment for yourself. It seems rather obvious, but when in doubt, ask someone who clearly knows what's what—preferably a staff member.

One way to avoid confusion when you first start out is to take advantage of new-member orientations. During these orientations, a staff member takes you through each workout apparatus and shows you how to adjust it to your level of skill and your specific physique. In addition, many gyms offer a workout log with each setting and adjustment recorded on a card to help guide you during future visits. You can consider this a road map to terrain that will soon become as familiar to you as your own backyard.

Similarly, you shouldn't be shy when it comes time to ask someone to be your spotter. (A spotter is someone who stands by to help you control the weight should you reach failure in the middle of a repetition.) This ensures you don't get stuck under a weight that's too heavy for you to remove. While a good spotter can help you squeeze out an extra repetition or two and help you get the most out of each exercise, the most important role a spotter plays is to ensure safety. One of the advantages of machines over freeweights is that machines are generally safer and, unless you want someone to help you squeeze out a few extra repetitions, don't require a spotter for the sake of safety.

When do you use a spotter?

◆ If you're doing an exercise you can't walk away from if you "fail" in the middle of a rep.

◆ If you want to get a little extra out of your workout, your spotter can help you do a few assisted reps instead of quitting as soon as you're out of gas.

◆ If you want to see how many repetitions you can get at a certain weight. Say, for example, you want to bench press 135 pounds 12 times but aren't confident you can do more than 10.

Finally, if a spotter isn't available, wait until a staff member or trusted fellow exerciser near you is available. In the meantime, don't just sit around; consider whether another exercise can do the trick by working the same muscle in a safer fashion. (As you'll see later, just about every freeweight exercise has a machine equivalent.)

The Collars

Collars are metal clips you put on the barbell to keep the plates from falling off the bar and onto a part of the human anatomy. They also ensure you don't break the plates, the floor, or anything else should they come flying off the bar due to recklessness and gravity.

Collars come in several types—some are squeezed on, others are clamped—but they all serve the same purpose. It doesn't really matter what type of collar you use as long as you use something. At some point in your gym career, you're likely to see some thick-chested guy lifting serious weight on the bench press without collars to secure the weight. With each bounce of the bar on his chest (a big no-no), the plates drift farther and farther toward the end of the barbell. This is a disaster in the making—especially if one of these behemoths is squatting 500 pounds. If one of the plates comes sliding off, it would be next to impossible to maintain balance. With that much weight on the shoulders, a serious injury to the lifter is inevitable, and anyone in the way of the plates is in trouble, too. (For whatever it's worth, we've rarely seen a woman shun collars on an exercise where it was necessary. If we have to shame the guys into proper collar use, so be it.)

Miss Manners Says ...

As a whole, human beings are a sensitive lot. The lack of civility in any locale—rush-hour traffic, waiting in line at the post office, or at your desk at work—is often quite upsetting. The gym is no exception. The importance of functioning politely and courteously in a setting in which you're likely to see many of the same faces day after day can't be stressed enough. Of course, the basic manners of normal society apply in the gym: no belching, passing gas, or other discourteous behavior is acceptable. However, you should know a few particular items of gym protocol to make everyone's life under the fitness roof more enjoyable—including your own.

Deidre and Joe know a hulking chap who was offended by a woman who refused to let him "work in" with her. (We discuss "working in" in a moment.) Here's a man who's worked out faithfully for more than 20 years, a man who has a shaved head and more muscles than most Rodin sculptures—in short, an intimidating figure—and yet her rude dismissal left him as wounded as a little boy excluded from a game of pickup basketball. "I can't believe that," he muttered over and over as he got madder and madder.

Civility is important—on the road, in the workplace, and in the gym.

We also know a man who often bellows so loud in the gym on his last few repetitions that one fears for anyone with a weak heart. Lest you think we're exaggerating, the roar is an obnoxious combination of a martial arts expert breaking bricks and an elephant orgy. Simply put, it's noise pollution.

Lightening the Load

Without question, one of the most common mistakes people make in the gym is leaving "their" weights on the bar when they're finished using them. Even if you're only using a pair of 10-pound weights, it's still rude to leave them.

Actually, the people irked most by this lack of gym courtesy are the staff members who work there. (Jonathan, who worked in gyms for 15 years, often did more lifting while cleaning up after gym members than in his own workouts.) People who regularly abuse their bit of gym protocol say they're "too busy" or "they plan to use the bar later in their workout." Sorry. Imagine a slender woman (who is probably just as busy) spending time hoisting 45-pound plates off a bar you just used. Be fair, and put back what you put on.

May I?

"Working in" with another person who is using the same piece of equipment you desire is one of the subtle practices in the gym you need to learn to feel at home. Let's say you want to do three sets of biceps curls on the biceps machine. If no one's waiting to use it, it's just fine to sit down and wait until you're ready to lift for your next set. If, however, someone's waiting to use the machine, it's common courtesy to ask him if he'd like to "work in" with you. (That's if he doesn't ask you first.) Unless you were just about to start your next set, proper gym etiquette dictates that you get off the equipment and allow the polite interloper to do a set. When he's finished a set, it's your turn. It often can seem like an inconvenience, but working in with someone ensures you don't dawdle between sets, which means you're likely to get a better workout. In the spirit of cooperation, it's a good idea to replace the pin at the weight the other person was using. Ditto on the seat height if you moved it.

Wiping It Clean

Here's another bit of obvious advice that's often ignored: wipe your sweat off the piece of equipment you've just used. Surprisingly, it's a practice that's frequently ignored. It's standard practice to work out with a small towel, bandana, or piece of paper towel. Some people place the towel between them and the seat or bench they're up against. Some just wipe it down after they're done. As long as the sweat is gone, either way is just fine.

The "sweating-on-the-equipment" phenomenon can be a touchy one, and some people clearly go overboard, audibly sighing as they wipe the very machine you've just thoroughly toweled off. Our experience is to let them do the extra housework and hope they get to a therapist who can help them deal with their intense reaction to the thought of someone else's perspiration.

Keep It Clean

Gyms have their own unique aroma. People sweat when they lift weights; run on treadmills; ride stationary bikes; and toil away on stair climbers, VersaClimbers, and rowing and cross-country ski machines. Just writing about it is enough to make one break into a cold sweat. All this sweat can turn a poorly maintained gym into a very, how shall we say, *pungent* environment. Most gyms, however, wash their machines with aromatic cleaning fluid as well as vacuum and scour the locker rooms.

Sweating is basic to a gym, but don't push your luck by wearing workout gear you've worn 3 days in a row. This is a good way to earn nicknames like "The Stinky Guy." And it's not advisable if you're planning to run for political office. In fact, wearing foul clothes will …

◆ Make it difficult to build friendships—at least friends with a sense of smell.

◆ Make finding a spotter tougher than finding Godot.

◆ Make you the topic of gym gossip.

◆ Make it highly unlikely someone will work in with you.

Of course, as we just said, this is a gym, not an opera house. The idea is to go there and sweat. And although no one expects you to leave smelling like a daisy, it's important that you and your clothing at least start out nose-friendly. If you haven't showered in 45 hours, avoid sleeveless shirts and please don't use the gym as the place to find out if your new deodorant's 48-hour guarantee really works.

The Least You Need to Know

◆ If you've been sick or injured or haven't exercised in years, get a physical before embarking on a new exercise regimen.

◆ Haven't been sick in years? Take the PAR-Q before you hit the gym.

◆ Once you've received medical clearance, ailments such as diabetes and asthma shouldn't hold you back.

◆ Fortify your brittle bones, tricky knee, and bad back with a well-designed strength-training regimen.

◆ Proper technique and attention to detail ensure your safety in the gym.

◆ How do you learn all the nuances of all of those machines? Ask. Learning what goes where is easier than you might think.

◆ Working in. Wiping off. Smelling clean. It's downright civilized.

In This Chapter

- ◆ Beginning a stretching program
- ◆ Stretching easy and breathing hard
- ◆ Learning how to stretch different muscles

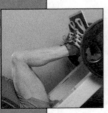
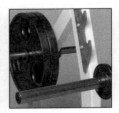
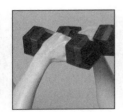
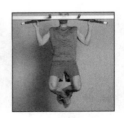
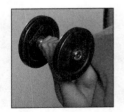
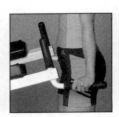

Chapter 4

Revving the Engine

Steve Ilg, a highly sought-after professional trainer and author of *The Winter Athlete* (Johnson Books, 1999), has been a nationally sponsored multisport athlete who has excelled in technical rock and ice climbing as well as Nordic skiing, cycling, and snowshoeing. He is also a yoga teacher and Joe Glickman's coach. Often when he's asked what the best way to stay flexible is, he replies, "Renounce your furniture. Learn the Asian squat and make use of it." It might sound absurd or amusing, but it makes sense. If you toss your chairs and tables, reduce the amount of desktop work you do, and eat your meals seated cross-legged on the floor, your lower back and hips will be far better off than the compressed lifestyle to which most of us are accustomed.

Although getting rid of your furniture might be good for your overall flexibility, it's likely to make your family and friends think you've either had a momentous religious experience or you're absconding with company funds and heading to Mexico. Assuming you keep your dining room set and La-Z-Boy lounger, you'll be well served to do the next best thing—embark on a regular stretching program.

"But I hate to stretch," you say. Sure, stretching can be tedious. Plus it hurts—at least when you first do it. And wine tastes like cough medicine the first dozen times you try it. However, the more you do it, the more limber your body becomes. Eventually, you'll get so accustomed and even fond of that self-lubricated sensation you'll crave it like a Frenchman does a fine Bordeaux.

If you're like the three of us—highly motivated fitness addicts leading busy lives—here's the way you probably think: *Time is precious, gotta get in and out of the gym as soon as possible.* However, let us assure you (and we're speaking from experience here), if you don't stretch and continue to work out, your body will rebel. Again, to quote Mr. Ilg, "More than a fitness quality that allows you to gain something, kinesthetic training enables you to release something that is already within." To borrow terminology from the martial arts: lifting weights is *hard* training; stretching is *soft*. Do both, and you're armed and dangerous.

It might sound dramatic, but almost more than anything else we tell you in this book, warming up and stretching are crucial if you're to stay healthy and achieve your fitness goals. Joe, who spends a lot of time crunching his 6-foot, 4-inch frame into a narrow, tippy kayak, suffered from a number of chronic, nagging injuries—the most pernicious being sciatica (a painful condition caused by compressing the sciatic nerve, which is located right behind the back pocket of your pants) in his left leg. Two weeks into his daily stretching routine, the pain virtually disappeared even though he continued paddling. Ditto for the achy feeling he experienced each morning in his lower back.

This chapter will guide you through the basics of warming up and stretching—the two most neglected aspects of the fitness game.

Warming Up: How Long Do I Stay on This Thing?

Years ago, runners and cyclists were taught to head out the door and hit the pavement at full stride—or at least to reach peak efficiency as fast as possible. (Hence the "no pain, no gain" theory.) This might work if you're a Marine in boot camp, but it's a great way to tweak cold muscles and ensure you're on the disabled list faster than you can say "illiotibial band syndrome." (IBS is a common running injury that affects the tissue that runs from the hip to the knee, often alleviated by stretching.) In time, virtually all aerobic athletes learned the virtue of a proper warm-up. And you should, too.

Warming up is the perfect catchall phrase for what you should do right after you enter the gym and change into your workout gear. Pick your favorite piece of aerobic equipment, and ease into an easy-to-maintain rhythm for approximately 10 minutes (although 5 minutes is better than nothing).

Here are our favorite machines to warm up on:

◆ **The Schwinn AirDyne.** This bicycle uses your arms as well as your legs.
◆ **The Concept II rowing machine.** This machine works your whole body.
◆ **The NordicTrack.** This machine simulates cross-country skiing. It's gentle on the joints but works your entire body.
◆ **A treadmill.** Put it on an easy setting, and tread lightly.
◆ **Elliptical trainer.** A great, nonimpact way to get the blood flowing. Those machines that use your arms as well as your legs are even better for a warm-up.

How fast should you go? That depends on how fit you are. In other words, if you're breathing heavily, you're going too fast. If your pulse is the same as it is while you're reading this book (unless you're reading it as you ride the exercise bike), you're going too slow. Your aim is to raise your body temperature as well as increase the blood flow to your muscles and joints. Just as you begin to sweat, it's time to move on to the next crucial stage of working out: stretching.

Hey, Stretch!

When you've finished warming up, head to the stretching area. Typically, this is a small, quiet room littered with mats. You'll know you're in the right place when you hear the loud "whoosh" of people exhaling.

Again, we can't overstress the importance of stretching to the quality of your workout as well as the quality of your life. Here's where you'll stretch each major muscle group. If the mere thought fills you with dread, it's all the more reason to suck it up and face your tight hamstrings.

Kids are naturally as loose as Gumby, but age and our sedentary lifestyles shorten our muscles. Think about it: you sit for hours each day and lie virtually motionless in bed for 8 or so hours at a time. Riding a bike, running, and clicking the keyboard of a computer shortens your muscles over the course of a lifetime. Without stretching, the natural length of a muscle is changed, which can lead to weakness and muscle imbalances, which can in turn lead to structural changes as you get older. Just thinking about it conjures up images of the Hunchback of Notre Dame.

The way to counteract this process is to stretch. Simply put, stretching maintains the flexibility that's compromised as we age. Flexibility is important in both everyday activities like turning your head before you make a left-hand turn onto the highway or bending over and picking up your 2-year-old child, as well as in athletic endeavors such as fielding a ground ball or shushing down the ski slopes without pulling a muscle.

In her work as a physical therapist, Deidre sees countless injuries that are directly related to decreased flexibility. Not surprisingly, virtually every one of these injured people complained about lower back pain. Care to guess how flexible they were? If you said "not very," you win a tube of Ben Gay. Once they were given a comprehensive stretching routine, their symptoms usually disappeared.

Now while Deidre told her patients to stretch like there was no tomorrow, she lifted weights each day and diligently skipped stretching herself. The result? During her

powerlifting career she suffered from chronic lower back pain. When she was evaluated, she was told that the flexibility of her lower back musculature was that of a 75-year-old driving instructor. When she began to stretch on a regular basis, this nagging injury receded into the background.

 Flex Facts

One of the best indicators of back pain and/or potential injury is the sit-and-reach test, in which a subject sits on the floor with straight legs and bends forward at the waist toward his or her toes. If your fingertips can't reach your toes, it's a sure sign you need to work on your hamstring and lower back flexibility. If you can't reach your knees, get to a yoga class.

Easy Does It

One of the reasons why motivated types like Jonathan and Joe postponed stretching for so long is that they viewed it as a cardio- or strength-training session. They saw it as a contest they waged with themselves (a particularly male condition known as *machismo*). This ability to try less hard is particularly irksome for these achievement types because they are so conditioned to believe that harder is better.

Here's where the *train hard, train soft* mindset must come in. The key words when it comes to flexibility training are *gradual* and *easy!* And as we discuss in a moment, the operative phrase is *belly breath.* Stretching consists of several fluid, graceful movements you do in concert with focused breathing. Done correctly, you should experience mild discomfort in one or more muscle groups, but not pain. If there is pain, there will not be gain.

Why? Inside your muscles are defense mechanisms called muscle spindles. The muscle spindles are quite sensitive to stretch. If your muscle stretches too far too fast, the muscle spindles pull back to shorten the muscle and prevent muscle or tendon damage. It's precisely because of this self-protective mechanism of the muscle spindles that it's so important to stretch correctly. Try too hard and you may actually end up with less flexibility rather than more.

To Do and Not to Do

Although most of us did it in high school gym class, bouncing while you stretch has gone the way of the beehive hairdo. It might have seemed like a good idea at the time, but we know much better these days.

If you bounce while stretching you're likely to engage those defensive mechanisms, or, worse yet, override them and pull a muscle. To state the obvious, don't bounce. It won't help your flexibility.

The three most important things to remember about basic stretching are …

1. Stretch to the point where you feel a gentle tension in the muscle. That sounds like a contradiction in terms, but it's really another way of saying you should ease into a mild state of discomfort well short of pain.

2. Hold the stretch for 20 to 30 seconds.

3. As you hold the stretch, breathe deeply, stretching just a little farther with each exhalation.

It seems somewhat silly to mention, but it's crucial to remember to breathe while you stretch. Breathing helps deliver fresh blood to your muscles. Get into the habit of practicing this deep-belly breathing. It will help you immensely when you lift weights. However, it's common practice to hold your breath as you move deeper into a stretch. Be mindful of this—it's a sign you're pushing too hard or are resistant to the task at hand—and return to your breath. Not only will this help you relax, it will allow you to stretch a little farther with each exhalation.

Deep breathing is not something we do naturally at rest. In fact, most of us breathe shallowly from the chest and don't use our *diaphragm*. Try this now: place one hand on your abdomen and one hand on your chest. Take a deep breath through your nose, and fill your abdomen with air (you should feel your hand rise with your abdomen). Complete the breath by filling your chest with air (you should feel your hand rise with your chest). Now exhale through your mouth, expelling air from your abdomen first, then your chest. Repeat this slowly 5 times. You may feel a little dizzy or light-headed, but that's normal because you're not used to such oxygenated air.

Of course, you're not going to place your hand on your abdomen or your chest while you stretch or lift weights. (It's challenging enough to lift with two hands, let alone one.) Instead, practice inhaling deeply through your nose and forcefully out through your mouth. Once you realize the positive effect this has on your stretching (not to mention your sense of well-being), it will be a standard part of your workout.

Now that we've convinced you of the importance of getting (and staying) limber, let's take a look at some of our favorite stretches. Starting a routine is a little like working your way into a great book. The first 50 pages may seem laborious, but once you get into it, you'll be hard pressed to put it down. Do the following for 2 weeks. You'll be surprised how grateful your stiff body feels.

Spot Me

For people who have scoliosis (sideways curvature of the spine), the torso stretch is a good stretch for the opposite side of the curvature. For example, for a left-sided scoliosis, stretch the right side.

Torso Stretch

Improving and maintaining a flexible trunk (torso) is extremely important for obvious reasons. If you've ever seen an elderly person (or someone with a back injury) bend down to pick up a piece of paper, you'll know what we mean. If your torso becomes stiff, simple tasks such as turning and reaching are compromised. In fact, you often hear of people who say they *threw out* their backs lifting a pot of water. In fact, that was merely the straw that broke the camel's back.

Here is what you need to do to stretch your torso:

1. Stand with your feet shoulder-width apart and toes pointed straight ahead.
2. Keep your knees bent slightly.
3. Place one hand on your hip for support while you extend your other arm up and over your head toward the ceiling.
4. Now slowly bend at your waist to the side where your hand rests on your hip.
5. Move slowly, gracefully, and continue to breathe.
6. Hold the stretch for 20 to 30 seconds.
7. Repeat on the other side.

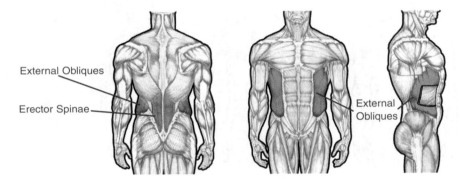

External Obliques

Erector Spinae

External Obliques

Torso stretch: muscles used.

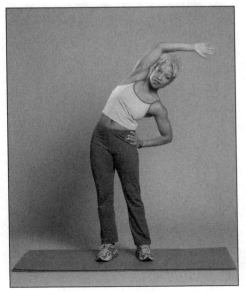

Torso stretch.

Pec Stretch

Here is what you need to do to stretch your pectoral muscles, the muscles of your chest that pull your arms forward:

1. Stand up or sit on a bench, and interlace your fingers behind your back.
2. Lift your arms up behind you until you feel a stretch in your arms, shoulders, and chest.
3. Keep your chest out and chin in.

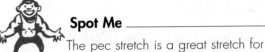

Spot Me

The pec stretch is a great stretch for people who suffer from asthma. Asthmatics tend to take on a forward chest posture, probably from difficulty breathing. This stretch opens up the chest muscles, freeing the muscles used for breathing.

This is a good stretch to do at any time, especially if you're at a desk and find yourself slumping.

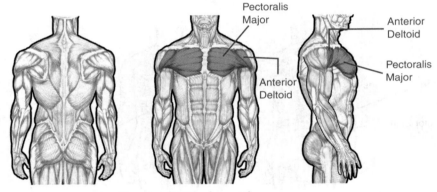

Pec stretch: Muscles used.

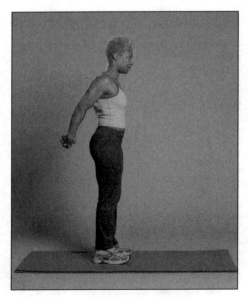

Pec stretch.

Spinal Twist

The spinal twist is great for limbering the muscles that align your spinal column. It also stretches the buttocks and hips. Here's how to do it:

1. Sit with your left leg straight on the floor.

2. Place your right foot flat on the floor over your outstretched left leg, and rest it to the outside of your left knee.

3. Place your left elbow on the outside of your upper right thigh just above your knee.

4. With your right hand resting behind you, slowly turn your head and look over your right shoulder. At the same time, rotate your upper body toward your right hand and arm.

5. During the stretch, use your left elbow to keep your right leg stationary with controlled pressure to the inside. As you turn your upper body, think of turning your hips in the same direction without lifting your hips off the floor. You should feel a stretch in your lower back and side of hip.

6. Hold for 20 to 30 seconds.

7. Breathe deeply. Repeat on the opposite side.

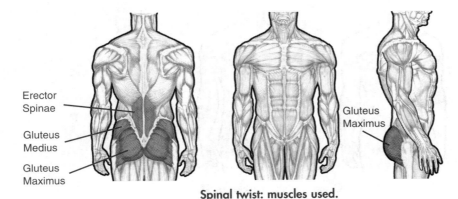

Erector Spinae

Gluteus Medius

Gluteus Maximus

Gluteus Maximus

Spinal twist: muscles used.

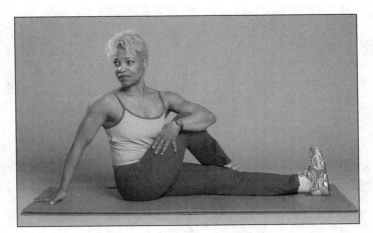

Spinal twist.

Groin Stretch

Tight groin muscles are a common source of strains in sports with sudden stops, starts, and turns. The groin is defined as the depression between the thigh and the trunk and consists primarily of tendons from your *adductor* muscles.

Here is what you need to do to stretch your groin muscles:

1. Sit with your spine straight.
2. Put the soles of your feet together, and grab your toes.

3. Bending from your hips, gently pull yourself forward until you feel a good stretch in your groin. Do not make the initial movement for the stretch from your head and shoulders; move from your hips. You may also feel a stretch in your lower back.
4. Hold for 20 to 30 seconds.

Bar Talk

The **adductor** muscles are the muscles that draw your leg in toward your body from an outward position.

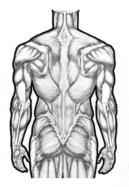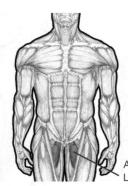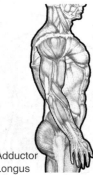

Adductor Longus

Groin stretch: muscles used.

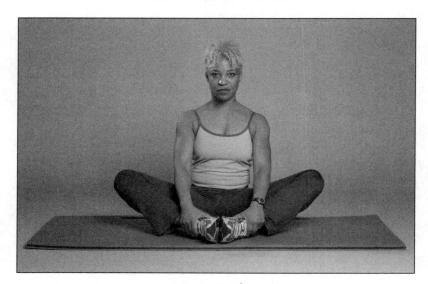

Groin stretch.

Quadriceps Stretch

The quadriceps (or "quads") are a group of four individual muscles—rectus femoris, vastus medialis, vastus lateralis, and vastus intermedius, if you must know—that attract so much attention when you walk around in shorts. They work together to straighten the knee. The rectus femoris is the only muscle of the four that crosses the hip. Your quads are the workhorses in activities such as running, stair climbing, squatting, and lunging.

To stretch these large muscles, do the following:

1. Stand near a wall for support.
2. Bend your right knee, and hold the top of your right foot with your left hand, gently pulling your heel toward your buttocks. Be sure your knee is pointing down toward the floor.
3. Keep your hips and shoulders level.
4. Hold for 20 to 30 seconds.
5. Breathe deeply throughout the stretch and then switch to the other leg.

Spot Me

The reason you hold your foot with your opposite hand is because the natural angle of the patellofemoral joint is not straight as you bend it; it turns inward with end-range flexion.

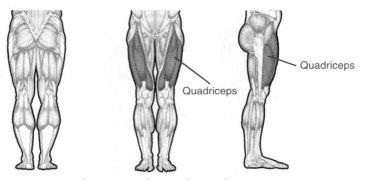

Quadriceps

Quadriceps

Quadriceps stretch: muscles used.

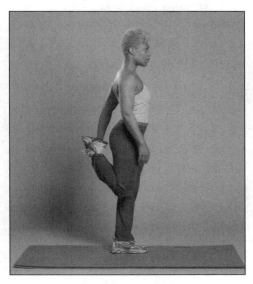

Quadriceps stretch.

Hamstring Stretch

The hamstrings are three individual muscles that oppose the quads—the biceps femoris, semitendinosus, and semimembranosus, for those of you keeping score at home. They work as a group to bend the knee and to straighten the hip. Tight hamstrings, a condition so common it sounds like the official name, can often contribute to low back pain. Keep them loose, and you'll feel like a new person.

Here is what you need to do to stretch your hamstrings:

1. Sit and straighten your right leg.
2. Place the sole of your left foot against the inside of your right thigh.

3. Slowly bend forward from your hips toward the foot of your outstretched leg until you feel a gentle stretch.
4. Hold for 20 to 30 seconds.
5. Once the initial discomfort has diminished, bend forward a bit more.
6. Hold for another 20 to 30 seconds.

Again, when the stretch becomes more comfortable, lean forward for the last time for another 20 to 30 seconds. Repeat this three-part move on your other leg. Remember to relax and focus on your breathing.

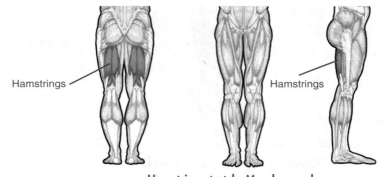

Hamstring stretch: Muscles used.

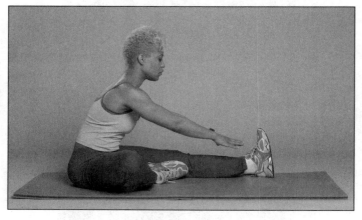

Hamstring stretch.

Hip Flexor Stretch

Next we have the hip flexor, as it is called in lay terms; to medical types it refers to the iliopsoas muscle, which flexes the hip. The hip flexors are instrumental in running, especially sprinting, as well as cycling and stair climbing.

Here is how you work your hip flexors:

1. Kneel on both knees.
2. Extend one leg forward so the knee of your forward leg forms a right angle directly over your ankle.
3. Gently lower the front of your hip downward so your back leg lies on the ground like an L.
4. Hold for 20 to 30 seconds.
5. Switch legs and work your other hip.

Be careful of this stretch if you have knee problems. Here's a fine alternative to that stretch:

1. Stand facing a support high enough that your hip and knee form a 90° angle.
2. Bend your left knee, and place your left foot on the support.
3. Your grounded foot should be pointed straight ahead.
4. Keeping your back straight, lean your hips forward until the heel of your standing foot lifts slightly from the floor.
5. You should feel a slight stretch in the front of your right hip. Hold for 20 to 30 seconds.
6. Repeat on your other leg.

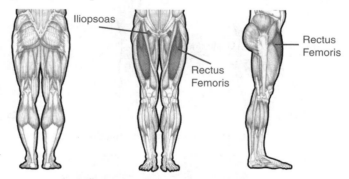

Hip flexor stretch: muscles used.

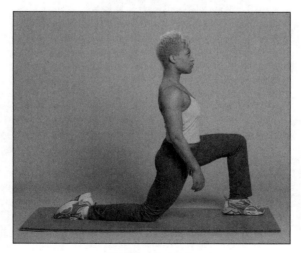

Hip flexor stretch.

Calf Stretch

To stretch your gastrocnemius (the calf to you and me), do the following:

1. Stand on a solid support, and lean forward against a wall.

2. Place one bent leg forward, and extend the other leg with a straight knee behind.

3. Slowly move your hips forward, keeping your lower back flat.

4. Be sure to keep the heel of your straight leg on the ground with your toes pointed straight ahead.

5. Hold for 20 to 30 seconds.

6. Don't bounce, be sure you breathe, and repeat on the other side.

Weight a Minute

For any stretch in which you have to bend your knee, be absolutely certain your knee doesn't "overshoot" your toe. The knee should never be farther forward than your toes; otherwise, there's too much stress on your knee.

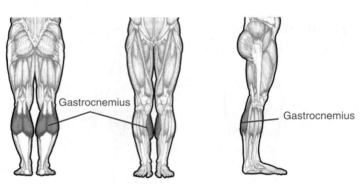

Gastrocnemius

Gastrocnemius

Gastrocnemius stretch: muscles used.

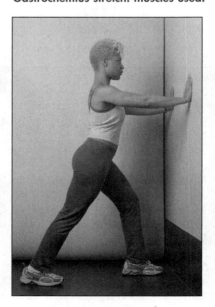

Gastrocnemius stretch.

Here's a wrinkle to the gastrocnemius stretch to work the deeper calf muscle as well as the Achilles tendon:

1. Assume the position we just described for the gastrocnemius stretch, but lower your hips downward as you slightly bend your back knee and bring it forward just a touch.

2. Be sure to keep your back flat.

3. Try to keep the heel of your back foot down.

4. Hold for 20 to 30 seconds.

5. Switch legs and stretch the other side.

Spot Me

Tight hamstrings and tight calves (also called the gastrocnemius) can be the source of a knee condition called *patellofemoral syndrome*. Symptoms can include pain during prolonged sitting and walking down stairs. Getting these muscles flexible can help alleviate this problem.

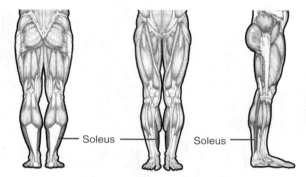

Soleus — Soleus —

Soleus stretch: muscles used.

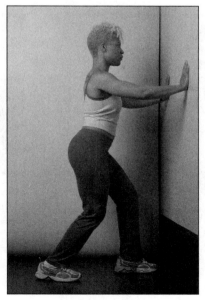

Soleus stretch.

Back and Hip Stretch

Here is what you need to do to stretch your lower back and the side of your hip:

1. Lie on your back, bend one knee at 90° and, with your opposite hand, pull that bent leg up and over your other leg, as shown in the following figure.

2. Turn your head to look toward the hand of the arm that's straight out with palm down (your head should be resting on the floor, not held up).

3. Placing the other hand on your thigh (just above your knee), pull your bent leg down toward the floor until you feel the right stretch feeling in your lower back and side of hip.

4. Keep your feet and ankles relaxed, and be sure the backs of your shoulders are flat on the floor.

5. Hold for 20 to 30 seconds, and repeat on the other side.

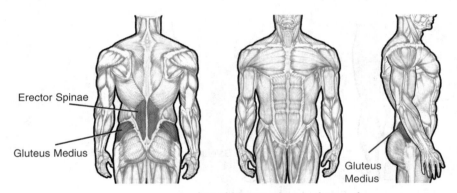

Erector Spinae

Gluteus Medius

Gluteus Medius

Back and hip stretch: muscles used.

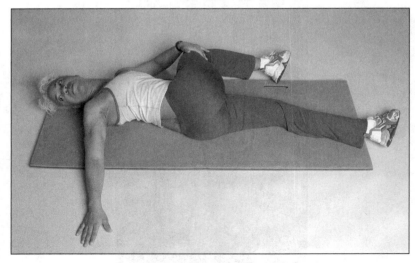

Lower back and side of hip stretch.

Here is what you need to do to stretch your middle back:

1. Stand and interlace your fingers out in front of you at shoulder height.

2. Turn your palms outward as you extend your arms forward as if pushing something away from you.

3. You should feel a stretch in your shoulders, middle of upper back, arms, hands, fingers, and wrists.

4. Hold for 20 to 30 seconds, and repeat twice.

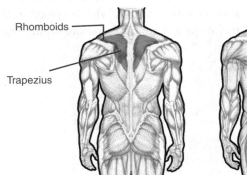
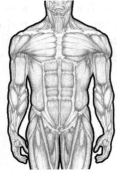
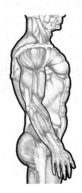

Rhomboids

Trapezius

Middle back stretch: muscles used.

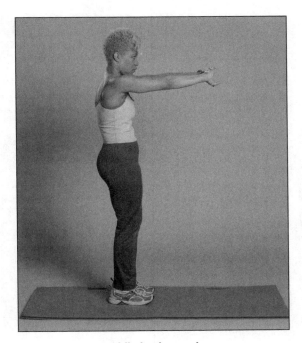

Middle back stretch.

Advanced Techniques

Static stretching is the most proven and safe method to increase flexibility, but you may come across other techniques in the gym. As we mentioned earlier, bouncing or ballistic stretching can be unsafe and ineffective, so we never advocate it. In Active Isolated (AI) stretching, a technique developed by Jim and Phil Wharton, the exerciser moves through a full range of motion by contracting the opposing muscle while stretching. The stretch is held for only a few seconds and then repeated.

Proprioceptive Neuromuscular Facilitation (PNF) is a technique more commonly used in therapeutic settings, but it has gained popularity among some personal trainers as well. It temporarily fools your defense mechanisms as you strongly contract the muscle you plan to stretch immediately before you do so.

Both AI and PNF are viable ways to stretch but should be treated with respect. A class or session with a trainer who is versed in these techniques is advisable before trying them.

The Least You Need to Know

◆ Age and a sedentary lifestyle make stretching a necessity.

◆ Stretch to the point where you feel a gentle tension in the muscle.

◆ Hold your stretches for at least 20 seconds.

◆ As you hold the stretch, breathe deeply, stretching just a little farther with each exhalation.

◆ Whether you're hustling after a bus or trying out for the Bolshoi Ballet, you'll feel and perform far better if you're limber from the waist down.

In This Part

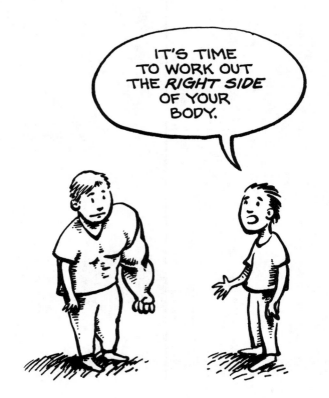

Part **2**

The Workout

It's funny how many people who start lifting have little or no idea what muscles they're working. "I want to work these things," they say, pointing to their deltoids. In Part 2, you'll find a complete list of weight-lifting exercises for your entire body. Each exercise is accompanied by photos and a thorough explanation of what to do. Why is it important to hold your elbows here or your knees there? Part 2, which tells you how and why, is your own personal trainer guiding you in print.

In This Chapter

- ◆ Learning the lingo
- ◆ Standing, bending, and sitting at your own risk
- ◆ Breathing big
- ◆ Remembering technique, technique, technique

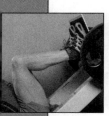 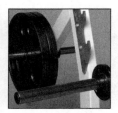 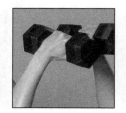 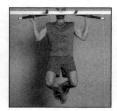 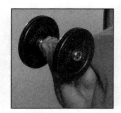 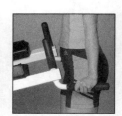

Chapter 5

Gluteus What?

It seems each sport, club, fraternity, family (or any other subset of society at large) has its own lingo, its own code words that the initiated use as shorthand. Cyclists "hammer," "jam," or "bonk"; street hoop junkies "slam," "dish," and do battle in "the paint." The gym, of course, has its own jargon. Words such as *pecs*, *quads*, and *lats* are tossed around like 5-pound barbells. These code words may sound like snippets of conversation between two narcotics cops, but they're actually abbreviated versions of the technical names for various body parts.

When Joe was a child, his uncle gave him an anatomy book he had used during medical school. Each page revealed another complete system: circulatory, nervous, muscular, and so on. As a child, pondering how these separate systems functioned as one filled him with wonder. Even as a busy adult, when you pause to consider the human body, only the most jaded mortician wouldn't be awed by the complexity of this amazing machine. Because you're going to be spending a fair bit of time working your muscles, we think it's important to be able to visualize what's going on beneath your epidermis. In fact, the better you understand how your muscles work, the easier it is to appreciate what we're talking about when it comes to particular exercises. In addition, gaining an appreciation for human anatomy might help ensure you maintain solid technique and not injure yourself.

In this chapter, we provide you with charts so you can familiarize yourself with the roughly 600 muscles that comprise your body, the very muscles you'll become intimately involved with in the near future.

Know What and Where It Is

Here's a partial list of common code words you'll hear at the gym:

◆ **Pecs (pectoralis major).** This is the body part Fabio made famous. In ancient Greece, soldiers were chided: "What do you want, a medal or pecs to pin it on?" The muscles of your chest, the pecs move the upper arm down and across the body.

◆ **Lats (latissimus dorsi).** Check out a world-class swimmer or kayaker from behind, and you'll see the sweeping expanse of muscle from the armpit to just above the waist that resembles a highly agitated cobra. The lats pull the upper arm back and down.

◆ **Quads (quadriceps).** From the waist up, Jonathan looks like a fairly normal athletic citizen. (Of course, looks can be deceiving.) However, from the waist down, he looks a bit like two loaves of bread with too much yeast. Why? As a cyclist who averages 5,000 miles a year, his quads are his biggest allies. The quads' main function is straightening the knee.

◆ **Hams or hammys (hamstrings).** Look at any Olympic sprinter's muscular legs for an example of what hamstrings can look like. Hamstrings, which are made up of three separate muscles that run from just beneath the backside to the back of the knee and are responsible for bending the knee, are as inflated as a side of beef in most of these guys. In fact, all superior sprinters and NFL running backs and anyone else who regularly needs a burst of speed have these sweeping, sculpted strands of muscle.

◆ **Bi's (biceps).** Large biceps (guns), the muscle that bunches up into a ball between your elbow and shoulder, are the classic symbol of masculine strength. What do Arnold, Vin Deisel, and Mr. Clean have in common? Big biceps! Without them, the tattoo business would be in dire straits. The biceps are to the arms what the hamstrings are to the legs—they bend your elbow.

◆ **Tri's (triceps).** The opposing muscle to the more famous biceps, triceps push while the biceps pull. This lopsided triangle of muscle on the posterior side of your upper arm is most visible when you do a push-up. The job of the triceps is to straighten your elbow.

◆ **Traps (trapezius).** If you've ever seen Mike Tyson sans shirt, you're likely to have noticed these two Brahma bull–like lumps that sprout from under his ears and connect to the tops of his shoulders. These pronounced loaves of muscle help shrug your shoulders and pull your shoulder blades together.

◆ **Delts (deltoids).** Atlas shrugged them, and we call them delts. It's the shoulder muscle, a large triangle-shaped muscle that covers the joint and serves to raise the arm laterally.

Flex Facts

The word *deltoid* is derived from the Greek word *delta*, which means "triangle." Take a look at a well-developed pair of delts, and you'll see why.

◆ **Abs (rectus abdominis).** Also known as the tummy, gut, and stomach—which actually is a misnomer—your abdominals run from the lower rim of the rib cage to the pelvis. Your stomach is the organ that digests your food. Well-developed abdominals (a washboard stomach) à la

Bruce Lee not only look great, but they will increase your athletic potency tenfold.

◆ **Glutes (gluteus maximus).** Buttocks, tush, backside, derriere, and many more are synonyms for this old trusted friend. Once developed, these oft-neglected muscles provide lots of *oomph* for forward propulsion.

Here's a nuance of gym vernacular you should know about. Typically, when someone is asked what body parts he's working on a particular day, the answer is something like "chest and back, shoulders and arms," and so on. Rarely will you hear someone say, "I'm working my pecs and delts." However, when lifters refer to a particular body part, they more often than not use the abbreviated Latin names we've just mentioned. For example, "Wow, your lats are huge." Or "Your abs are ripped." Or "Your quads look like a chicken that needs a tan." (Just for the record: the first two are highly complimentary; the latter is a solid insult.)

The following is a chart of the muscles of the front (anterior aspect) and back (posterior aspect) of the body.

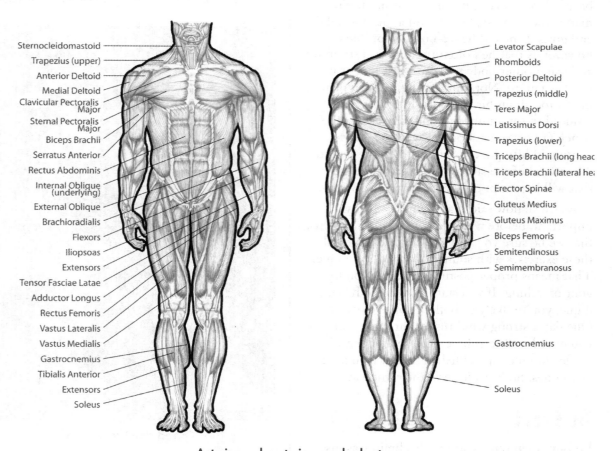

Anterior muscle chart labels:
- Sternocleidomastoid
- Trapezius (upper)
- Anterior Deltoid
- Medial Deltoid
- Clavicular Pectoralis Major
- Sternal Pectoralis Major
- Biceps Brachii
- Serratus Anterior
- Rectus Abdominis
- Internal Oblique (underlying)
- External Oblique
- Brachioradialis
- Flexors
- Iliopsoas
- Extensors
- Tensor Fasciae Latae
- Adductor Longus
- Rectus Femoris
- Vastus Lateralis
- Vastus Medialis
- Gastrocnemius
- Tibialis Anterior
- Extensors
- Soleus

Posterior muscle chart labels:
- Levator Scapulae
- Rhomboids
- Posterior Deltoid
- Trapezius (middle)
- Teres Major
- Latissimus Dorsi
- Trapezius (lower)
- Triceps Brachii (long head)
- Triceps Brachii (lateral head)
- Erector Spinae
- Gluteus Medius
- Gluteus Maximus
- Biceps Femoris
- Semitendinosus
- Semimembranosus
- Gastrocnemius
- Soleus

Anterior and posterior muscle chart.

Walking Tall

At first glance, lifting weights is less risky than, say, waterskiing or rock climbing. All you need to do—once you join a gym—is walk in and start lifting. Herein lies the rub. In sports such as waterskiing, the risky elements are obvious: fast boat, hard water, big ouch. Assuming you don't drop a barbell on your forehead, the risk in weight lifting tends to be cumulative—the proverbial drop in a bucket that one day overflows and stains the carpet.

Take a chap we know at the gym—a short, bearded, muscular guy who trains hard. No matter the exercise, he piles on a lot of weight and gives it the old heave-ho. The problem, however, is that he's often twisting and straining and using other body parts to assist him as he reaches failure. Not long ago he was complaining to Joe about his sore left shoulder. He reduced the amount of weight he used on the bench (a notorious shoulder wanker), but he continued lifting like a man paid by the pound. The moral of the story? Arthroscopic surgery that will keep him out of the gym for 6 weeks.

As we've now said many times, it's very important, before we have you hoisting weights, that we be sure you will be able to execute all these exercises with sound form and technique. That means proper posture and attention to your breathing. If you start using shoddy technique, you're likely to build a house of cards. One day a strong wind rushes through, and you're reduced to rubble. And remember, it's harder to unlearn bad habits than it is to learn good ones. So learn it here, the right way.

Be Erect

Woody Allen once said that his brain was his "second favorite organ." Most men would probably agree, but when it comes to your overall health, your back is the most important body part you have, principally because it's the core

to which everything (muscles, nerves, etc.) is attached. As a private-practice physical therapist, Deidre saw many ailing patients who complained about back pain after a particularly strenuous gym workout. The biggest culprit? Lousy technique.

Try this exercise:

1. Stand against a wall so the back of your head and your buttocks are flush against it.

2. Now take one step forward, tighten your stomach muscles, and keep your buttocks in the same position—almost as though you have a tail tucked between your legs.

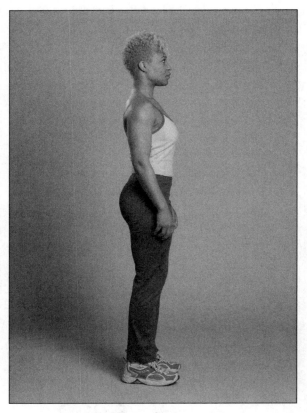

Correct standing posture.

This is the position you should maintain while performing any standing weight-lifting exercises. At first you might feel like a

Buckingham Palace guard or an English school-marm, but once you get used to feeling comfortable like this, you'll be righting a lot of postural wrongs. The bottom line here is that when you're properly aligned, your abdominal muscles help protect your back and decrease excessive *lordosis*, a condition that can be a source of back pain. Bad posture is enough to injure your back, but start stressing your skeleton with weights and the plot only thickens.

Bar Talk _____

Lordosis refers to the natural inward curve of the lumbar or lower spine. In some people, especially those with potbellies, the curve is greater than normal and can be the source of back pain.

Sitting Bull

As we have mentioned, an excessive amount of sitting can wreak havoc on your skeletal structure. Let's set the record straight: we aren't anti-sitting—in fact, we sat throughout the writing of this book. However, too many of us sit too much of the time—for hours at work, in front of the television, in the car to Grandmother's house, and more. Most often we are sitting in chairs that are improperly fitted for us and, if you're a desk jockey who talks on the phone a lot, this unnatural position adds another wrinkle to the bad posture formula. Toss in a good dose of stress—"What, the order won't be here till Tuesday?"—and you understand why massage is such a thriving business.

Twenty-five percent of the patients in Deidre's physical therapy practice had back (upper and lower), shoulder, or neck pain from sitting either too much or improperly. How can such a passive activity as sitting cause so many problems? Here are some reasons:

- When we sit, there's more pressure on the lumbar spine than when we stand.
- When we slouch in a chair or couch, the *erector spinae* muscles are overstretched for an extended period of time, which weakens them. Weak muscles tend to spasm because they have to work harder to perform simple tasks such as sitting straight.
- Serious slouchers crane their necks forward to see what's in front of them. This puts significant pressure on your *cervical spine* and can cause weakness, spasms, and headaches.

Bar Talk _____

The **erector spinae** muscles run along either side of the spine and are instrumental in good sitting posture. The **cervical spine** is the part of your spine that attaches your head to your body. When someone says, "He's lost his head," he's indirectly talking about the cervical spine. It is composed of the first seven vertebrae from the base of your skull (C1) to the largest protrusion you can feel (C7).

Here's more good news: poor posture can also cause shoulder problems. How? Try this: slouch in a chair and raise your arms overhead. Now sit up straight. Notice a difference in your range of motion? Slouching does not allow proper engagement of your rotator cuff muscles, which can weaken them over time and lead to problems such as *impingement syndrome*. Impingement syndrome is a painful shoulder condition that can be caused by several factors, including a weak rotator cuff. As you raise your arm, an arc of pain radiates in your shoulder. Often strengthening the weak muscles in the area resolves the problem.

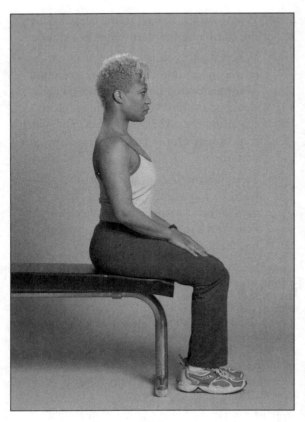

Proper sitting posture.

Bend Right

Let's assume for a moment that after reading about the various skeletal maladies you haven't quit your job, sold your furniture, and moved to a yoga ashram to find postural enlightenment. Instead, let's hope you at least recognize the importance of sitting up correctly and the subsequent importance of stretching. Unfortunately for the poor unsuspecting weight lifter, another danger is lurking in the shadowy recesses of your neighborhood gym: improper bending—probably the number-one cause of lower back pain. Luckily, it's also the most preventable.

Our backs are built to withstand a tremendous amount of pressure. Our spines, flexible pieces of architectural genius, act as shock absorbers to counteract forces that occur from walking, running, skipping, hopping, driving, sky diving, weight lifting—well, you get the point. However, our backs are not built to withstand the rigors of bending all day long, especially when picking up heavy objects.

If you continually bend the spine of a book in the opposite direction it was meant to go, it eventually weakens and breaks. This is more or less what happens with your spine when you continually use your back incorrectly, day after day, year after year. In her private practice, Deidre heard countless times, "I just bent over to pick up my shoe, and my back gave out." Well, that may be the way it seemed, but that's not the way it happened.

"How," you may ask, "should I bend if not from my back?" Ironically, most of us know how to bend correctly because we have ample practice doing so when we have a stiff and sore back. When your back is ailing, you be sure you use your hips and your knees to lower your body to the ground and to raise yourself back up again. Your legs have the largest muscle groups in the body for a reason.

All this has considerable practical application to the time you spend in the gym, because you have to bend to pick up weights and you have to bend to put them back. To state the obvious: it is very important that you do this correctly.

Try this exercise:

1. Stand against a wall with your feet shoulder-width apart, roughly 6 inches from the wall.
2. Begin to slowly slide down the wall while bending your knees.
3. Now step away from the wall and lower yourself into a deep knee bend while keeping your back straight.

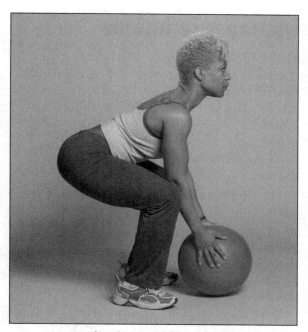

Proper bending and lifting technique.

This is how you should use your back at all times, whether picking up a gum wrapper or a 45-pound barbell.

In and Out

Joe's coach, Steve Ilg, is a big proponent of training an athlete's mind, body, and spirit. Peppered throughout his training schedules are small reminders that pay huge dividends. Here's one to keep in mind whenever you train: "Spine erect, breath full and deep, yet soft."

Breathing properly allows you to merge with the activity at hand. This might sound like a line from *Kung Fu*, but it's one of the most important techniques you can use. Why? The link that connects the body and the mind—a hard-to-describe but easily felt connection—is the breath. Not only will this help you lift more and better, it is also a key way to alleviate boredom in the gym.

Conversely, breathing shallowly or even holding your breath is like working out while wearing a corset. Done under extreme stress, holding your breath can cause you to black out by cutting off oxygen to your brain. And you increase the chance of having a stroke by aneurysm.

Try this exercise:

1. Inhale deeply through your nose and then exhale through your mouth. Repeat this five times. (If you're not used to breathing from your diaphragm, you may feel a little dizzy.)
2. Now, sit in a chair with your arms by your side.
3. Inhale through your nose.
4. Now raise your arms until they are shoulder-level and exhale through your mouth.
5. Next, lower your arms while inhaling through your nose.

This little exercise is a way to introduce you to how you would be breathing in the gym while performing shoulder raises.

Spot Me

When you're lifting weights, remember to forcefully exhale in the concentric or power phase. This will ensure that you breathe through the most difficult part of the exercise when the tendency is to hold your breath. To help you to remember, keep this in mind: exhale on effort.

Up Three, Down Three

Earlier, we referred to the use of momentum as a way to "cheat" when lifting (read: men eager to lift more than they should). This use of body English (cheating) makes the exercise easier and puts a ton of stress on various joints in your body. It may help you lift more weight, but this jerkiness ensures that you're not giving the specific muscle group proper attention. By using the technique of "up three and down three," you will effectively remove momentum from the gym and put it back in Physics 101 where it belongs.

Here's how this simple but effective technique works:

1. Stand with your arms by your side. While bending your elbows, count "one-and-a," "two-and-a," "three-and-a." By the end of "three-and-a," your elbows should be fully bent. Pause for one count at the fully contracted position.

2. Now reverse the process and straighten your elbows. As you do so, count "one-and-a," "two-and-a," "three-and-a." By the end of "three-and-a," your elbows should be straight. (We recommend you do this silently unless you're a bandleader or kindergarten teacher.)

This count helps you to move slowly, establish a good rhythm, and ensure that you're depending entirely on the muscles you should be working.

Here's a quick checklist of reminders you should take with you on each trip to the gym:

❑ Perform all standing exercises with proper standing posture.

❑ Perform all sitting exercises with proper sitting posture.

❑ Bend from your hips and knees, not your back.

❑ Breathe properly, in through your nose and out through your mouth.

❑ Remember the count—3 seconds on the positive phase of the lift, a 1-second pause, and 3 for the negative.

Improper Technique

Here's a solid bit of irony. After reading the preceding information, you may decide that it's easier to perform exercises improperly, and you're probably right. When you enlist other muscles to assist you, hold your breath, or use momentum to your advantage, the exercise becomes easier but at a cost—safety and effectiveness.

We want to make this very clear so when you see incorrect technique you know it. Furthermore, we don't care who's doing it—the huge guy with the bulging biceps or the trainer, yes the trainer, who is showing an exercise to a novice who doesn't know a dumbbell from a doorbell.

We know a trainer who advises all his clients improperly. In fact, when Deidre hears him tell clients to "throw your back" into a biceps exercise or recommend they perform leg extensions at breakneck speed, she's tempted to walk over and hand the client her physical therapy business card. The majority of trainers know their stuff, but this is a good reminder that you shouldn't take everything a trainer teaches you as gospel. Don't be afraid to challenge them and have them explain their thought process if it's something you don't understand. If we question our doctors, we can certainly question health club trainers.

Weight a Minute

Oftentimes, using bad form makes it easy to hoist more weight, but not without a price. The extra weight may make you feel stronger, but it won't really strengthen your muscles. Worse still, bad form makes any exercise more dangerous.

Cheers

Water, water everywhere, but alas, few of us drink enough of the stuff. This is even more applicable for people who work out. The key fact to remember is that by the time you're thirsty, your body is already dehydrated. The trick is to head off that thirsty fiend at the pass and stay topped off in the first place.

If you notice that you're lethargic or sore or experience muscle cramps or irritability after a particularly hard workout, the odds are you're dehydrated. It's recommended that you drink at least 80 ounces of water per day even if you don't exercise that day. Remember, now that you're increasing your activity level, you must drink more water to maintain proper hydration.

We don't expect you to keep track of how many ounces of water you consume, but an easy way to tell if you are hydrated is to note the color of your urine. If you're well hydrated, it will be virtually colorless (unless you take vitamins). If it's a concentrated yellow and you don't take vitamins—drink up, mate!

You can do as we say, or learn the hard way. Take Deidre, the powerlifter who preached the virtues of stretching but who hardly stretched until she was so compromised she had to to get out of bed in the morning. Before training for the New York City Marathon in 1999, she still wasn't convinced she needed to drink more than a few glasses of water a day—until she completed a 9-mile run that left her wiped out with fatigue and muscle soreness for 2 days. After several demonstrative vows of "liquid repentance," she heeded this traditional hydro warning and drank the appropriate amount of water for a week before her next long run. Much to her surprise, she felt much better during and after the run. As you no doubt know, there's nothing worse than the zeal of a recent convert!

The Least You Need to Know

◆ Proper attention to posture—sitting, standing, and bending—is essential.

◆ Understanding the importance of proper breathing further ensures the mind/body connection.

◆ Remember that by the time you're thirsty, your body is already dehydrated; the trick is to stay topped off in the first place.

In This Chapter

- ◆ Understanding physiology fact and fiction
- ◆ Determining how long, how much, and how often
- ◆ Learning what's in a rep

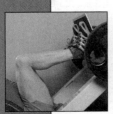 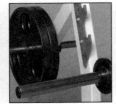 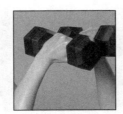 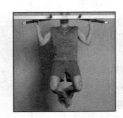 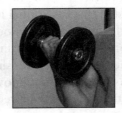 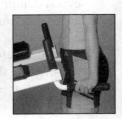

Chapter 6

Now What?

Strength training is part art, part science, and part luck. The science is how to lift and when. On the physiological front, we know a lot about what happens when you follow specific training guidelines. The art is applying this knowledge to your body. For example: how hard do you lift? Are you able to back off when you're tired and push harder when you're stuck at a plateau? Does your diet complement your fitness goals or sabotage them? And a host of other factors govern the way one progresses in the game of fitness. The luck part revolves around one word: *genetics*.

In other words, a lot of variables surround a lifting program—some you can obviously control, some you can't. In this chapter, we discuss the various x-factors involved so you have a better understanding of how you can best progress in the gym. For example, here's a question that continually stumps people: why will two people who work out together, doing virtually the same routines, progress at different rates? Read on.

That Was Intense!

Having said that, of all the variables in your lifting program, how hard you work—let's call it the *intensity factor*—is the single most important one you can control. In this chapter, we give you plenty of tips on how to safely increase this intensity factor so you get better results faster.

Of course, some variables aren't under your control: age, gender, muscle fiber types, and a few other genetically determined variables play a major role in your strength development. We'll talk about what they are and how you can work with them instead of getting frustrated and giving up.

It's Quality, Not Quantity

There are no real differences between the muscle fibers of men and those of women. On a pound-for-pound basis, women are capable of becoming as strong as men. (When Deidre competed as a powerlifter, on a pound-for-pound scale she routinely outlifted most of the men at the meets.) However, because men tend to be larger and have a greater percentage of lean tissue (lower percentage of body fat), men generally have greater strength potential. Dr. Wayne Westcott put it best: men are stronger than women due to muscle quantity, not muscle quality. There are differences between the sexes, but the methods used to train women need not be any different than those used for men. And in fact, the glut of *women's exercise* programs arises more from a marketing angle than from genuine need.

How Long?

Consider this scenario: identical twins Tim and Tom are seated on opposite sides of a seesaw. If Tim sits all the way at the end while Tom sits 3 feet from the end, Tom will be airborne despite the fact they are exactly the same size. It's an issue of simple physics.

Now picture two workout partners who have been training together for 1 year. Let's say they're doing biceps curls. If both lifters are using the same weight and lifting with the same intensity, one may outlift the other by a substantial margin. Why? Again, it's physics, because the lifter with the shorter arms will have much less work to do. Clearly, there's no reason for the longer-armed lifter to alter his training program—and reducing your arm length is far too drastic a course to follow—but it would explain why the shorter-armed chap is progressing at a faster rate.

Now here's one you've probably not spent a lot of time pondering: tendon length.

Remember that tendons attach muscle to bone. Let's consider the biceps curl again to show how tendon length can affect strength. The biceps muscle runs from the shoulder to a point just below the elbow. Sparing you the physiological details, you might be interested to know that if your tendon attaches farther from the elbow, it's analogous to being at the far end of the seesaw. Similarly, an attachment closer to the joint is analogous to being in the middle.

Of course, there's nothing you can do about where your tendons attach to the bones; however, this will help you understand why you and your training partners don't always progress at the same rate. Because many people get discouraged when their partners progress faster, it's good to know why not all arms were created equal. Other than the fact that everyone is different, here's the good news: lift diligently and intelligently, and you'll get stronger. In short, you'll be building the body you've always dreamed about.

Fiber Types

If you went to the lab to construct the perfect weight lifter, you'd use lots of fast-twitch muscle fibers (they're the kind capable of the greatest gains in size and strength), short arms and legs, and long tendons. When 6-footer Jonathan accompanied Deidre to her powerlifting meets, he felt like Kareem Abdul-Jabbar at a jockey convention. At a bicycle race, he looks like one of the herd. (This may explain why he went into bicycle racing rather than competitive lifting.) Nevertheless, he lifts diligently to improve his cycling performance. On the other hand, Deidre, who carries 122 pounds of sculpted muscle on her 5-foot, 3-inch frame, has the ideal muscle type and body for hoisting prodigious amounts of weight. Did she have to train like a Trojan to become a world champion? Definitively yes. Could she have been a comparatively good cyclist or basketball player? Smart money says no.

Your next question might be: if you can't change these things, why even bother discussing them? For the simple fact that knowing about these variables can help prevent unnecessary frustration in the weight room. As we mentioned earlier, everyone can get stronger from weight lifting, but each person responds differently, even if the stimulus is the same.

Now that you know about some of the things we can't alter, let's talk about some of the things we can. Luckily, no matter what your genetics, height, or body type are, the body is an amazing machine that adapts beautifully when called upon. If you run a lot, your legs will respond; if you swim or kayak a lot, the upper body snaps to attention. The same is true of lifting weights: lift right, lift often, and the gains are there to be had.

Get With the Program

Although there are unyielding universal truths when it comes to developing a strength-training program, it's just common sense to tailor your routine to you—and not some prototypical lifter who may have different goals, time constraints, and so forth.

Starting in Chapter 7, we give you a variety of exercises to work all your major muscle groups. Don't know how to awaken your dormant latissimus dorsi? No problem—we offer step-by-step instructions. And in Chapter 18,

we give you suggestions about which exercises are most appropriate for you given your specific goals. After all, if you want to improve your 10K running time, buffing up your biceps isn't time well spent. Strong hamstrings—well, that's a muscle of a different color.

For now, let's go over some of the fundamental aspects of a sound training routine.

What to Do?

For virtually every body part we discuss, we show you a few exercises. For every exercise we show you, there are usually at least two or three more—some good, some not so good—you could do instead. In most cases, these exercises are interchangeable. They're not really all that different. The most important thing to do is to be sure you train all your major muscle groups and train them in the right order. Right order? Yes. As we mentioned earlier, if, for example, you train your biceps first, your arms are likely to be too tired to offer proper assistance when you work your back or shoulders. As a rule, it's best to work the larger muscles first and work in descending size order. If you were going to hit all your major muscle groups on a particular day, you'd start with, say, your hips and legs and move down the list:

1. Hips and legs
2. Back
3. Chest
4. Shoulders
5. Biceps
6. Triceps
7. Abdominals

No, that's not written in stone—for instance, there's no real problem with switching chest and back or biceps and triceps—but it's a good guideline.

Schedule

When it comes to weight lifting, more is not always better. For instance, your initial temptation may be to take your ambitious mind and eager muscles to the gym as often as possible, but that strategy can actually work against you. Again, one essential key is to know when to work out and when to rest. Too much of one or the other, and you've upset the apple cart.

Keep in mind that as you lift, you're actually fatiguing and wearing down the muscle tissue. It's during the recovery process that your muscles actually grow bigger and stronger. So you should never train the same muscles on consecutive days; it's actually counterproductive.

That's where a *split routine* comes in. This is a program in which you train different muscles on different days. So although you might lift on consecutive days—chest, shoulders, and triceps on Monday; legs, back, and biceps on Tuesday—you'll be using different muscles each day. Not only does this allow ample time for your muscles to recover, it means you'll be doing fewer exercises on any given day. This prevents burnout, allows you to spend less time lifting on each visit, and means you'll be able to work more intensely on the exercises you do. Right now, don't sweat the particulars, because we'll talk lots more about split routines in Chapter 16.

Bar Talk

A **split routine** is a strength-training program in which you divide your body's muscles into two or more groups. On the first day of a split routine you train muscle groups A and B; the following day it's on to groups C and D.

At the other end of the "too many" spectrum, if you train too infrequently, the strength gains you made in one session will be lost by the next. Even if you do the best routine in the world on January 1 and little or no training until February 1, the result would be minimal at best in the strength gains department. That should come as no surprise, but we hear people who lift twice a month lament the fact that they're not making much progress.

So what is the ideal frequency? That varies from individual to individual and has a lot to do with how hard each training session is. Here's another immutable rule to note: a hard workout will require more recovery time than an easy one.

Individual strengths and weaknesses aside, two workouts per week is good; three may be better. Whenever possible, we advise beginners to aim for three workouts. If you manage to do two, fine; however, if you're shooting for two, the tendency is that you miss one and compromise your gains. There's another reason why three sessions may be better than two. Early in your workout life, one of our primary goals is to get your brain and body used to the exercises. At this stage we're less concerned with intensity than frequency. So don't worry about your body's ability to tolerate three workouts a week. Once you make going to the gym a regular part of your life—when your weight-lifting workout becomes part of your regular routine—we'll up the intensity and really start to see significant gains.

Reps

The repetition, or *rep*, is the basic unit of any weight-lifting program. Think of each rep as the nails a carpenter uses to hammer the studs of a house. Although you need to know the big picture, the walls will fall down if you don't pay proper attention to which nail goes where. Unless you first focus on each and every rep, other variables such as how many reps per set, how many sets per exercise, and the choice of exercise don't really matter.

How Fast?

Because it's quite important that each and every rep be performed with proper technique, let's do a quick rep check review.

A good guideline to follow while you're performing that perfect rep is to count to 3 during the positive or concentric phase, hold for a count of 1, and count to 3 for the negative or eccentric phase. By controlling the speed, you accomplish a couple productive things:

◆ First (and foremost), you maximize your safety and minimize the stress on your joints.

◆ You also ensure that momentum is a non-factor, which means you stress the muscles as much as possible and get the best bang for your buck.

◆ Finally, by keeping constant form for every rep of every workout, you're able to measure your progress.

For those of us who are goal-oriented (which tends to be just about everyone who works out regularly) or for those who just like to know that something is working, doing each rep as we just described is vital.

Spot Me _____
A good way to gauge if you're doing an exercise too fast is to try to stop at various points along the range of motion. Done correctly, you should be able to stop on a dime without momentum carrying you farther than you want.

Consider the following scenario. On January 1, you do a biceps curl with 15-pound dumbbells and are able to do 11 repetitions in a 3-1-3 cadence with textbook-perfect form. If by March 1 you're up to 13 reps, with the same weight and form, clearly you have made progress. On the other hand, if you never pay any attention to anything other than how much weight you hoist and how many reps you've done, an increase in how many reps you do could be due to changes in form rather than strength gains. This type of approach highlights our "lift to gain strength, not demonstrate strength" philosophy. It's not the best way to impress your musclehead friends in the gym, but it's a great way to get strong and healthy while staying injury-free.

Weight a Minute _____
It's important to perform each repetition in a slow, controlled fashion. This not only ensures that the exercise is effective, but it also minimizes the chance of orthopedic injury.

How Many Reps?

Now that we've established how you should perform each rep, let's examine how many reps you should do in each set. Walking around your local gym, you're likely to hear all sorts of different theories. Odds are that few, if any, are based on fact. Many will be based on refined analytical thinking that goes something like this: _Big Bob does sets of 25 for each exercise, and he's bigger than anybody else in the joint. That must be the way to go._ Or: _I read in a bodybuilding magazine that Ms. Olympia never does more than 5 reps per set, so that's what I do._ Again, how big and strong you get is largely a factor of genetics. Just because Bob the Bruiser is as broad as a barn door doesn't mean you will be, too. In fact, some guys out there get big just by looking at a dumbbell rack.

Wander around the gym a little longer and you're also likely to hear another bit of misinformation that goes something like this: using high weight with low reps builds bulk, but low weight and high reps helps build definition. Sometimes people will even tell you that lifting like that will actually elongate the muscle. Not so!

Here's the scoop. First of all, despite what you may hear from misguided trainers or in Pilates class, your muscle isn't going to get any longer by lifting weights—it attaches to a tendon, which attaches to a bone, and that's that. As for the notion that high reps will define or tone your muscles any more than low reps, wrong again. There are just no medical facts to substantiate such a statement. Too many other factors such as genetics and nutrition come into play; and besides, it's intensity, not the number of reps, that makes most of the difference.

Where this supposedly correct fact came from, we don't know. Perhaps it derives from the fact that a long set often produces a burning sensation in your muscles—flashback to Jane Fonda in a leotard encouraging you to "feel the burn"—but that's just due to an increase in the *lactic acid* in your bloodstream, and doesn't indicate that fat is being burned. Muscles look defined when there's a minimal layer of fat covering them. It's as simple as that. So the question remains: how many reps should you do? For most exercises, a range of 10 to 12 repetitions at a 3-second, pause, 3-second cadence is appropriate. When you can perform more than 12 well-executed reps at a given weight, it's time to up the weight by about 5 percent. The last rep of the set should always be a challenge—a noble effort we refer to as *elegant failure*.

Flex Facts

Muscular fatigue and a burning sensation during strenuous exercise are often due to a high concentration of lactic acid, which accumulates in the blood when the energy demands of an exercise exceed the supply or utilization rate of oxygen.

How Many Sets?

Once again, ask five so-called experts about the optimal number of reps to do, and you're likely to get five different answers. In fact, this question produces quite a bit of controversy; controversy, we must add, that's based on fiction rather than on fact.

Traditionally, lifters have performed 2 or 3 sets per exercise, though often you hear about people doing as many as 5 or 6. However, if you read the copious number of studies on the subject, most of them seem to indicate that 1 set (yes, 1 set!) can be just as effective as and far more efficient than doing multiple sets. By effective, we mean you can get every bit as strong. By efficient, we mean you can gain strength in a fraction of the time. If you use that extra time to do your cardiovascular training, to stretch, or to practice your sport, you're upping your fitness quotient twofold.

When Jonathan played junior varsity basketball at Hunter College, he observed many of the varsity players spending several hours a day in the weight room. Although they got plenty strong, they also shot a measly 65 percent from the foul line. Those players probably would have been much better served by cutting their lifting time in half and practicing their shooting.

Now, we're not saying you can't or won't get strong from 2, 3, or more sets per exercise—of course, you will—just that you can probably get as strong from 1 set, too. At the very least, 1 set is far more *efficient* than multiple sets. Again, whether you do 1 set or 10, the most important thing to keep in mind is that the last repetition of any set should be difficult. That's why it's important to avoid what we call the *magic number syndrome*. This occurs when people stop at a given number of reps (usually 10, 12, or 15) even though they've got a lot of gas left in the tank. If you reach your tenth rep and you can do another rep or two without sacrificing form or safety, do it. Remember that you're not a Swiss watch but an evolving work in progress.

How Much Weight?

How much weight should you lift? This question is probably asked more than any other question in weight lifting.

Now that we've established that a range of 10 to 12 reps is ideal for most exercises, we need to find the weight that will allow you to do that many without compromising your form. As we said before, early on your goal is to learn to do the exercises with the proper technique. In this initial phase of your lifting life, you should err on the side of caution when picking a weight to start with. Generally, the larger the muscle, the more weight you can handle. And as you'll quickly learn, you can move more weight with your legs than with your arms.

In Chapter 7, we begin to give you step-by-step instructions on how to actually perform these exercises. When you get started with each of them, begin with the lightest weight possible. If it's a machine, set it to 1 plate to get the feel for it and then add a little more. Right now we want you to focus on technique without worrying about completing the lift. For exercises that require dumbbells, use relatively light ones to accomplish the same aim. And for exercises with a barbell, try using the Olympic bar without weight, or even a lighter one if necessary.

In any event, be sure not to strain or push too hard during your first few workouts. After you get the feel of things, you can gradually start to increase the weight during the next few workouts. Be patient. Increase the weight a little each time until you find a weight that will be challenging by the tenth or eleventh rep. When you've found that weight, stay with it until you can do 12 good reps. When you can do 12 solid reps without straining a vital organ, it's time to increase the weight. When you bump up the weight, try for about a 5 percent increase. Adding that extra weight should make reaching 10 a challenge again.

Here's another issue to keep in mind: if you've been lifting for 6 months and find you're unable to perform 12 reps even though you did so last week, don't worry. The key is form, concentration, and intensity. As long as you reach elegant failure on your ninth, tenth, or eleventh rep, you're making progress. Lack of sleep, stress, and myriad other factors impact how you feel on any given day, so cut yourself some slack as long as you're working hard.

How Much Rest?

The amount of rest to take between exercises is as fundamental a concern as any other, but for some reason it is the one issue often overlooked. For example, most gym veterans can tell you how much weight they use and how many reps they do for any exercise, but few pay much attention to how much rest they take between sets.

From a physiological point of view, there's no real reason to take more than 3 minutes between sets. By that time, your ATP (remember, ATP is your body's source of immediate energy) is about 99 percent replenished and your body is as ready as it's going to be. From a practical point of view, there's no reason for a beginning lifter to wait that long between sets. Two minutes allows your muscles ample time to recover and gives a workout partner time to change the weight and do a set, without wasting undue time.

We don't want to make working out into a stressful bit of time management, but you should be aware that when you're not thinking about time, 2 minutes flies by. In fact, very often people have *brief* chats between sets that last anywhere from 4 to 15 minutes. Ask them how long they take between sets, and they assume it's only a few minutes. Before you know it, the workout that should take you 45 minutes to an hour has stretched to 1½ hours. As a result, early on at least, it's good to time yourself between sets. After you find a rhythm, your body will know the appropriate amount of rest to take.

For certain advanced programs such as circuit training (see Chapter 16), supersets (see Chapter 15), bodybuilding, or powerlifting (see Chapter 17), we vary the recommended rest interval. But for now, let's stick with 2 minutes.

Spotter, Please

Remember, a spotter is someone who is ready to help the lifter in case he or she can't complete a lift. As someone who has chosen to lift a heavy object—often over your precious head or neck—it's your responsibility to be sure you have a spotter whenever you're doing an exercise that may jeopardize your health and welfare. Probably the two most important exercises to have a spotter for when you're using free-weights are the squat (see Chapter 7) or bench press (see Chapter 9), but they're not the only ones. Again, if you can't lift the weight, you're in serious trouble.

Even when you're using a machine or doing freeweight exercises where your safety isn't jeopardized by the absence of a spotter, a helping hand can help you get more out of an exercise.

How? Everyone has exercises he or she finds particularly difficult. Let's say for you it's shoulder presses. (For an illustration, see Chapter 10.) Oftentimes, just having someone stand next to you provides the extra motivation to focus and finish the set with good form and maximum effort. Also, a spotter can help you get a few extra reps out of any exercise by offering the barest assistance. We've had spotters who provided invaluable help simply by nudging the weight with two fingers.

As the lifter, it's your responsibility to tell the spotter what you're going to do. Let him or her know how many reps you're hoping to do,

if you want a spot on the *lift off* (when you first pick the weight off the stand), and so on. It's also your job to never give up on a lift. Jonathan has helped spot powerlifters bench pressing more than 400 pounds. He couldn't lift close to that much by himself, but as long as the lifter doesn't *bail out* on the lift, he'll never have to. In fact, even if the bruising powerlifter can't moose out that last rep, as long as he gives it his best effort, Jonathan only has to help out with the last few pounds.

Sooner or later, you'll be asked to switch places and act as a spotter. In that case, it's your job to ensure the lifter's safety. Here's the key: never agree to do something you can't. And if you're not sure what's expected of you, ask. A good spotter is like a good baseball umpire—as unobtrusive as possible. Aside from an inattentive one, an overanxious spotter is the next biggest sinner. After you've ensured that the lifter doesn't drop 200 pounds on his esophagus, the spotter's job is to be sure the weight keeps moving with as little assistance as possible. Remember, you're doing the lifter a disservice if you provide *too much* assistance.

If you see the weight stop moving, give it a little nudge. (On most exercises that use a barbell, you're usually best off by lifting the bar itself. In the case of exercises that use dumbbells, it's usually preferable to nudge the lifter's elbows.) After you've done it a few times, you'll get the hang of it. The most important things to keep in mind are to always pay attention, don't jump in too soon, and stay close enough to the lifter to help out whenever needed.

Now that you understand the various x-factors of weight training, let's move on and learn some specific exercises.

The Least You Need to Know

◆ Understanding why no two lifters are alike should clear up a lot of questions as well as potential frustration you may feel.

◆ The anatomy of a repetition is of the utmost importance.

◆ The nitty-gritty of a strength-training program includes how many reps, how many sets, and how much weight.

◆ Offering assistance to your fellow lifters is a standard part of gym etiquette.

In This Chapter

- ◆ Understanding what's what
- ◆ Building your legs with two great freeweight exercises
- ◆ Getting buffer gams with seven leg-machine exercises

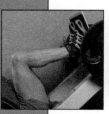
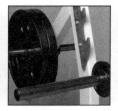
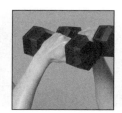
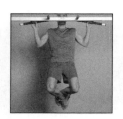
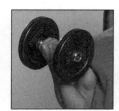
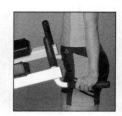

Chapter 7

Below the Waist

Okay, anatomy fans. What's the largest group of muscles in your body? Lats? Wrong. Pecs? Nope. Abdominals? Sorry. In fact, the largest muscles you have are located below your waist. When most people think of their legs, they think of the muscles in two major groups: upper and lower or thighs and calves. There is, of course, a lot more going on in those sturdy legs of yours. So you know what we're talking about when we recommend the exercises that follow, here's a quick tour of Leg World.

One of these muscle groups is the *gluteus maximus*, or glutes, a wide band of muscle that covers your entire butt area. If you've ridden a horse too long or cycled for hours at a time, these are the muscles that doth protest too much. They are also the muscles that are featured in all those salacious jean ads. The glutes, of course, can do more than sell pants. Their primary function is to extend your legs from your hips when your leg is bent. In other words, when you're running for the bus.

Located opposite your glutes are your *hip flexors*. Although several muscles contribute to the act of hip flexion, the largest is called the *iliopsoas*. These muscles don't receive much attention. In fact, in all our years of going to the gym we've never heard someone say, "Hey, nice iliopsoas." (We think this is a shame, but there's not much we can do about it.)

The iliopsoas is a strong muscle that doesn't need much concentrated work because it receives quite a bit of work on a daily basis with walking, running, and climbing stairs. In fact, because we tend to sit so much, it is the muscle that is often too tight. As a result, this muscle is usually better served by being stretched than by being strengthened. If it becomes too tight, this tricky muscle that runs from the lumbar spine to the inside of the uppermost part of the long bone in the thigh (femur) can pull your pelvis forward and put stress on your lumbar spine. The result? Serious lower back pain.

On the sides of your hips are the hip abductors, the main one being the *gluteus medius.* This muscle works to move your leg away from your body—while pushing off during inline skating, for example. Their companions, located on the inner part of the thigh, are the *adductors*, which draw your leg toward your body.

The big boys in the band are the *quadriceps*, or quads. These muscles span the entire front part of your leg. If you're an NFL running back or a professional cyclist, odds are your quads are like large loaves of bread. The quads are comprised of four muscles (hence the name *quad*riceps) that work to straighten your lower leg from a bent position. One of them, the *rectus femoris*, crosses the hip joint and works to bend as well as flex the hip.

Opposite the quadriceps are your *hamstrings*, which cover the entire posterior aspect of your upper leg. The hamstrings are actually three muscles that work in concert to perform two actions: to extend your leg from your hip when your leg is straight, and to bend your lower leg from the straight position.

Finally, your *calves* are the muscles located near the bottom of your legs. One of them is the *gastrocnemius* (or gastroc). This diamond-shaped muscle works to push you up on your toes. The other muscle, the *soleus*, is deeper and comes into play when your knees are bent and you need to lift your heel. The third muscle, located on your shin in the front of your leg, is called the *tibialis anterior*. This is the muscle that rears its ugly head when you come down with a case of shin splints. It functions to lift your toes from the floor. Think back when you've been speeding down the highway and seen flashing lights in your rearview mirror. The muscle that pulls your lead foot off the gas pedal is the tibialis anterior. In fact, the next time you're stopped by a cop for speeding, tell the officer you have chronically tight tibialis anteriors. If that doesn't work, hope you have a pregnant woman in the car.

What's the Point?

We hear comments like these all the time: "I'm a swimmer—why do I need strong leg muscles?" Or "I cycle a lot, so I don't need to work my legs." Or "I'm a runner and don't want to do leg exercises because my legs will get too big"—or any number of other faulty lines of reasoning.

Here are good reasons why lifting weights with your legs will serve you well:

◆ Strong leg muscles are the key to injury prevention in sports from cycling to running. In fact, weak leg muscles are the number-one reason runners are unable to complete proper training for a marathon or finish the race itself.

◆ Strong legs help your performance on the field. For example, some people think a pitcher such as Roger Clemens can throw a baseball nearly 100 miles per hour because he has an exceptional right arm. Of course he does, but much of his power is generated by his powerful hips and thighs.

◆ Strong muscles protect your hip, knee, and ankle joints from a lifetime of stress—from running, jumping, and going up and down stairs.

◆ They look good when you wear shorts. Similarly, just think about how weird it looks to have a great upper body and itty-bitty legs.

◆ For the elderly, keeping the legs strong is important for balance, walking moderate to long distances, and moving from a sitting to a standing position.

Now that we've convinced you you need strong legs, let's show you how to get them.

In general, most of the lower body exercises we recommend for you use machines; however, two freeweight exercises can contribute to an extremely effective lower body routine. These exercises—the squat and the lunge—involve not only your legs, but your entire body to stabilize you during the performance of the lift. Oh yeah, one sobering note: both are difficult.

Squat

Ah, the beloved and dreaded squat. The squat, a lower-body exercise that requires you to shoulder a barbell and literally squat, is a great way to strengthen your legs. When the 122-pound Deidre was powerlifting at the world-class level, she was able to do 8 repetitions with 185 pounds. In competition, her personal record is 330 pounds. Although no sane person (at least no sane 122-pound person) will attempt to do that much weight, the point is that squatting is a demanding exercise. Despite its incredible payback, it is extremely important that you pay strict attention to your form—and that you never lift more than you can safely handle. We omit squats from beginning programs, but we keep them in the arsenal for when you get the hang of things.

A few other words of warning: work with a spotter whenever possible, and be sure you're good and warmed up. Squatting when your legs are stiff is a great way to court injury. If a spotter isn't around, be sure to use an apparatus that's designed for squatting. A cage, such as the one pictured in the following figures, is designed to catch you if you can't get up from the squatting position.

Flex Facts

The squat is one of the three lifts competitive powerlifters do. (More on powerlifting in Chapter 17.) Using supportive gear such as wraps, suits, and belts (stuff we discussed in Chapter 1), competitive lifters bend farther down than parallel to the ground—the depth we recommend for you.

Here is how you properly perform a squat:

1. Stand underneath the barbell with your feet slightly wider than shoulder-width apart.

2. With your arms holding the barbell with a grip about 6 to 8 inches from your shoulders, lift the barbell off the rack.

3. Take one step backward so you don't hit the racks as you squat, and keep your toes pointed slightly outward.

4. Keeping your back straight, begin to bend your knees until your thighs are parallel to the floor. Don't squat deeper. However, if you squat too little you're not maximizing the benefits of the exercise—remember that a greater range of motion ensures full strength gains.

5. Return to your starting position.

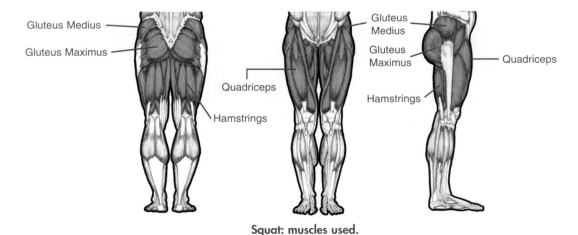

Squat: muscles used.

When performing a squat, **don't:**

◆ Lean forward as you squat.

◆ Squat without a spotter or safety rack.

◆ Place the bar across your neck.

Spot Me

Although some trainers consider it safer to do a *quarter squat* where you only bend to about 45°, we question whether that's the case. When you cut the range of motion that far, there's a tendency to greatly increase the weight that's used, which puts much more stress on your back.

Do:

◆ Keep your abdominals tight.

◆ Keep your weight on your heels, not on your toes.

◆ Maintain an upright posture.

◆ Place the bar across your upper back.

Spot Me

To work on keeping your back straight and your chest up, you may want to practice squatting with a broomstick.

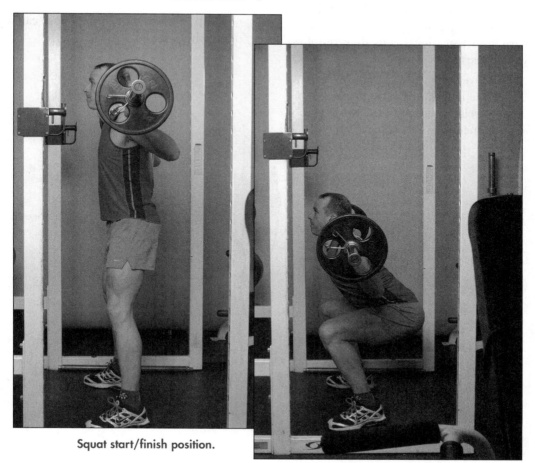

Squat start/finish position.

Squat middle position.

Lunge

Lunges use the same muscles as squats do. However, you don't need nearly as much weight because you're exercising one leg at a time. Lunges also require more concentration. Space out, and you're likely to lose your balance. Whether you do lunges or squats is a personal preference, because you don't need to do both. Deidre eschews lunges because she'd rather get both legs done at the same time. Because Jonathan has a strength deficit between his right and left legs, he does them a lot more for the left leg.

Here is how you properly perform a lunge:

1. While holding a dumbbell in each hand (palms facing your outer thighs), stand with your feet slightly less than shoulder-width apart.

2. Now move your right leg approximately one stride length in front of your left. The exercise is called *lunge*, but it is more aptly named *controlled lunge*.

3. Bend your right and left knees until your right thigh is parallel to the ground.

4. Return to the starting position. Repeat with the left leg.

When performing a lunge, **don't:**

◆ Lean forward.

◆ Let your knee pass forward of your big toe in the middle position.

Do:

◆ Keep your abdominals tight and back straight.

◆ Keep your torso upright.

Keep in mind that this exercise can also be done with a barbell.

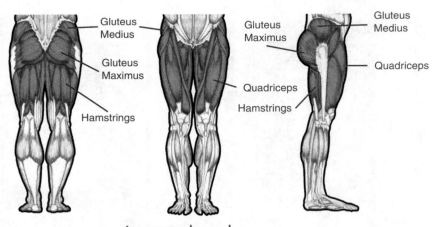

Lunge: muscles used.

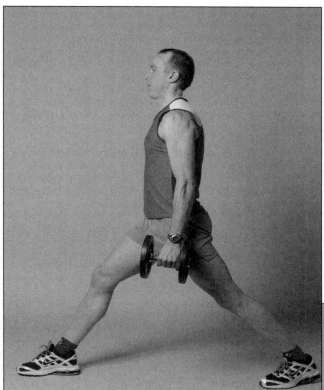

Lunge start/finish position.

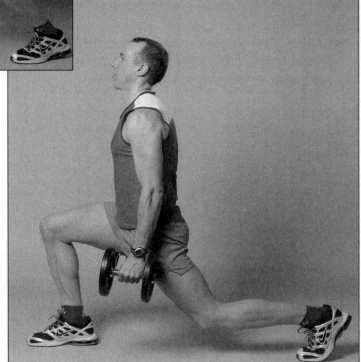

Lunge middle position.

Leg Press

The leg-press machine is one of our favorites because you can safely work both legs at the same time even while using a lot of weight. However, don't be fooled just because it's a machine; we know of people who have injured both their back and their ribs. How? For some reason, people have a tendency to load on a lot of weight. By stacking on too many big plates, the overloaded sled comes crashing down as soon as they release the brake. The obvious point? Don't add more weight than you can safely control for 10 to 12 repetitions.

The keys to a safe workout on the leg-press machine are as follows:

◆ Select an appropriate amount of weight you can safely do on your own.

◆ Bring the sled down slowly. Maintain control.

◆ Don't allow your lower back to rise up off the seat pad. If this happens, you are bringing your knees too close to your chest.

Weight a Minute _____

This exercise may be contraindicated for people with hyperextended (excessive backward bend) knees.

Here is how you properly perform a leg press:

1. Position yourself on the machine, and place your feet on the sled approximately shoulder-width apart.
2. Point your toes outward slightly.
3. Grasp the handles on either side of the seat.
4. Disengage the brake, and slowly lower the sled until your knees are bent to 90° or until your lower back comes off the sled.
5. Pause and slowly return to the starting position.

When performing a leg press, **don't:**

◆ Lock out or snap your knees at the top of the movement.

◆ Arch your back.

◆ Allow your buttocks to lift off the seat.

Do:

◆ Keep your abdominals tight.

◆ Bear weight on the midfoot to heel portion of your feet, not your toes.

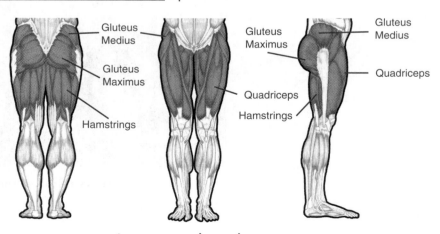

Leg press: muscles used.

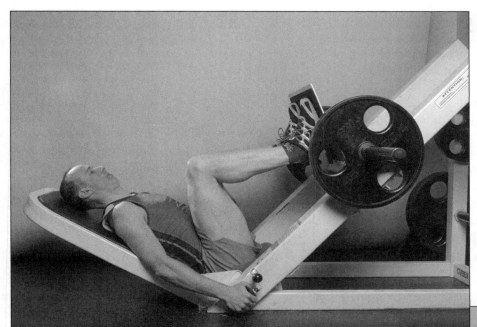

Leg press start/finish position.

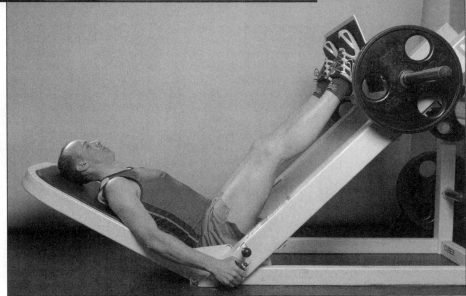

Leg press middle position.

Leg Extensions

Want quads like Lance Armstrong's? Do leg extensions. (Of course, it would help if you rode a bicycle 500 miles a week.) Okay, perhaps you won't build the legs of a Tour de France champion, but done diligently, leg extensions are among the best ways to build powerful upper thighs. Be very careful not to do more weight than you can handle for 10 solid repetitions. If you overdo it on this machine, you could end up with patellar tendinitis (an inflammation of the tendon just below the knee caused by overuse).

Here is how you properly perform a leg extension:

1. Sit down with your back against the back pad, and position your shins behind the lower leg pad.
2. Grasp the handles on either side of the seat.
3. Straighten your lower legs as high as possible.
4. Return under control to the initial starting position.

When performing a leg extension, **don't**:

◆ Jerk your legs up rapidly.
◆ Allow the weights being lifted to slam down against the weight stack between repetitions.
◆ Lock out or snap your legs straight.
◆ Swing your trunk back and forth.

Do:

◆ Keep your back against the back pad.
◆ Focus on your quads.

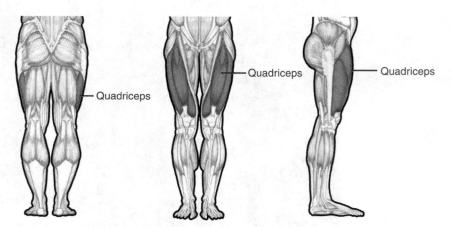

Leg extension: muscles used.

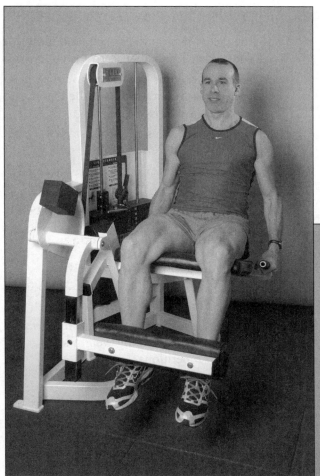

Leg extension start/finish position.

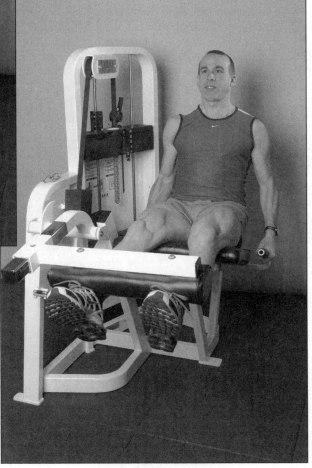

Leg extension middle position.

Leg Curls

Leg curls are to your hamstrings what leg extensions are to your quads. Because muscular balance is so essential, it's important to build both your quads and your hams so one doesn't overwhelm the other. Again, remember to stretch your hamstrings before doing this exercise.

Weight a Minute

Leg curls are not recommended for people with low back pain or hyperextended knees. Some gyms have a leg curl machine on which you sit rather than lie down that would be more appropriate for people suffering from back pain. For people who have hyperextended knees, a standing leg curl machine would be better. If you don't have these options, do the following: for lower back pain, place towels beneath your abdomen to give your back support. For hyperextended knees, adjust the rotary arm so your knees are slightly bent.

Here is how you properly perform a leg curl:

1. Lie face down on the bench, and place your lower legs underneath the roller pads.
2. The tops of your kneecaps should be positioned just over the edge of the bench pad and not on the pad itself.
3. Grasp the handles on either side of the bench.
4. Pull your heels up as close to your buttocks as possible.
5. Slowly return to the initial starting position.

When performing a leg curl, **don't**:

◆ Arch your back or lift your pelvis.
◆ Lie with your head in the left- or right-side position. Rest on your forehead.
◆ Allow the weight stack being lifted to slam down on the remaining weight stack between repetitions.

Do:

◆ Be sure you attain an angle of 90° or less at the midposition.
◆ Keep your hips on the bench.

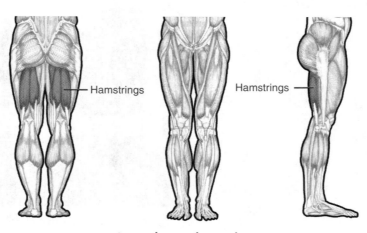

Leg curls: muscles used.

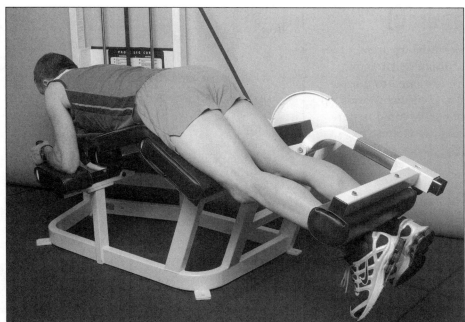

Leg curl start/finish position.

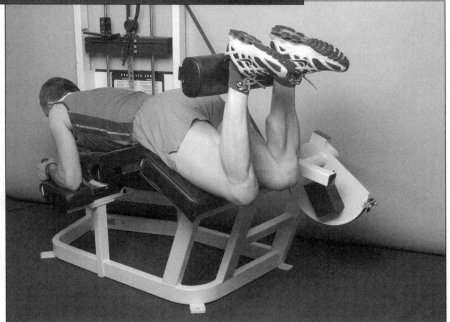

Leg curl middle position.

Calf Raises (Standing)

Much of your ability to continue to do even the most basic activities is due to muscular endurance. Muscular endurance is related to muscular strength. If you want to continue to walk up stairs with a spring in your step, you'd better begin to strengthen those gastroc muscles.

Here is how you properly perform a standing calf raise:

1. Stand on the bottom step so the balls of your feet are on the edge of the step and your heels extend over the edge.

2. Position your shoulders beneath the pads, and place your hands on either side of the pads.

3. Keeping your legs straight, rise up onto your toes as high as possible.

4. Return slowly to a position where your heels are hanging down as far as possible. This will ensure a good stretch.

When performing a standing calf raise, don't:

◆ Arch your back.
◆ Rock back and forth.
◆ Perform the exercise rapidly.

Do:

◆ Keep your abdominals tight and your back erect.
◆ Keep your legs straight.
◆ If it burns, you're doing it right.

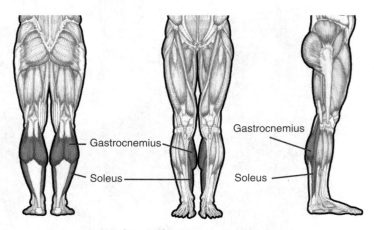

Standing calf raise: muscles used.

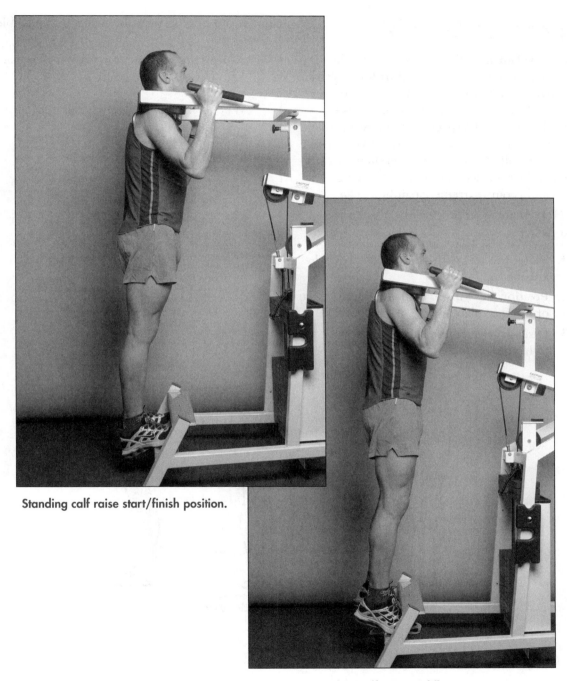

Standing calf raise start/finish position.

Standing calf raise middle position.

Calf Raises (Seated)

As we explained earlier, the soleus muscle is engaged while the knee is bent. It follows that the way to strengthen this muscle is to do so while the knees are bent. This muscle is extremely important, especially if you're a runner. It is a deep muscle (located close to your lower leg bone) called into play with endurance activities. If these muscles are weak, they fatigue and can become extremely painful.

Here is how you properly perform a seated calf raise:

1. Sit on the seat with your knees under the kneepads.
2. Position the balls of your feet on the edge of the foot plate.
3. Disengage the brake, allowing your heels to hang over the edge.
4. Rise up on your toes as high as possible.
5. Return slowly to a position where your heels are hanging down as far as possible to ensure a good stretch.

When performing a seated calf raise, **don't**:

◆ Rock back and forth.
◆ Perform the exercise rapidly.

Do:

◆ Keep your abdominals tight and your back erect.
◆ Remember, burn baby burn.

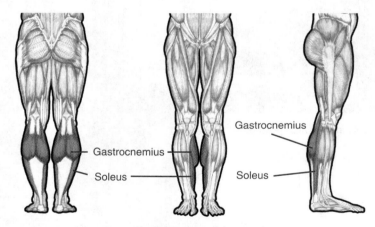

Seated calf raise: muscles used.

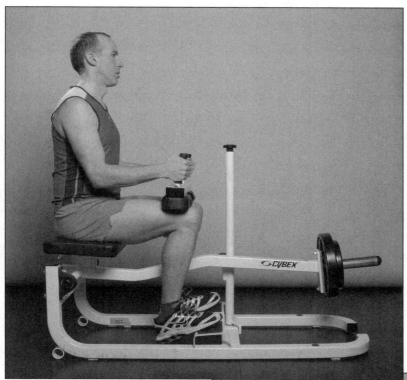

Seated calf raise start/finish
position.

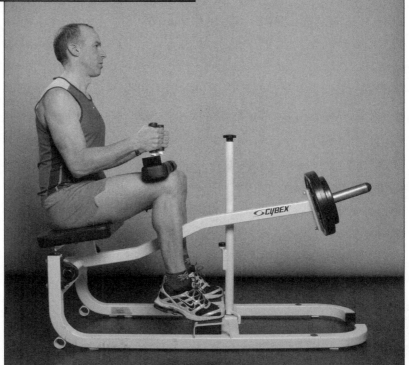

Seated calf raise middle position.

Hip Abduction

Because our muscles don't work in a vacuum, you don't really need to isolate your hip abductor muscles, because they are busy stabilizing and working while you're performing exercises such as squats and lunges. However, there is no harm done if you choose to isolate these muscles.

Here is how you properly perform a hip abduction:

1. Sit on the machine with your back against the back pad and your outer legs against the thigh pads.
2. Secure the belt if there is one.
3. Push your legs apart as far as possible by pushing against the thigh pads.
4. Return slowly to the initial starting position.

When performing a hip abduction, **don't**:

◆ Bend forward as you perform the exercise.
◆ Allow the weight stack to slam down on the remaining weight stack between repetitions.

Do:

◆ Keep your abdominals tight and your back erect.
◆ Keep your head and trunk against the back pad.

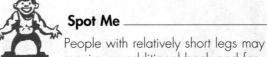

Spot Me

People with relatively short legs may require an additional back pad for this exercise.

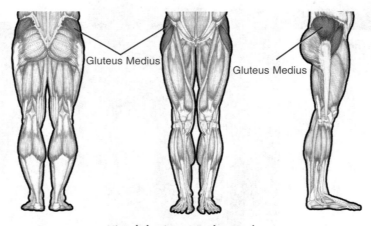

Gluteus Medius

Gluteus Medius

Hip abduction: muscles used.

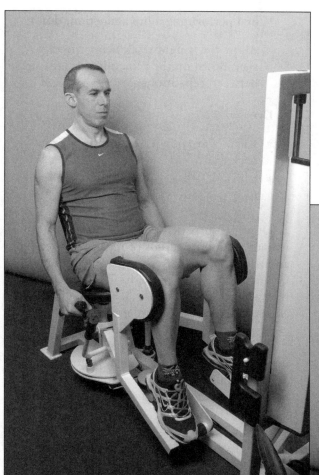

Hip abduction start/finish position.

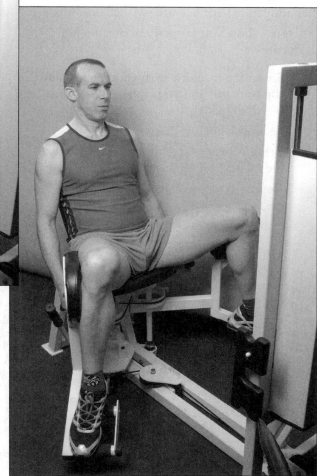

Hip abduction middle position.

Hip Adduction

Our muscles are not islands unto themselves; your adductors are working in conjunction with other muscles while doing squats, leg presses, or lunges. However, if you are involved in a sport that overstretches and/or overuses the adductors, you will definitely need to isolate them with these exercises. When Deidre powerlifted, she developed adductor tendonitis in both legs because she constantly overstretched her adductors with her wide-stance deadlifts.

Here is how you properly perform a hip adduction:

1. Sit on the machine with your back against the back pad and your inner legs against the thigh pads.
2. Secure the belt if there is one.
3. Bring your legs together as close as possible by pushing against the thigh pads.
4. Return slowly to the initial starting position.

When performing a hip adduction, **don't:**

◆ Allow the weight stack being lifted to slam down on the remaining weight stack between repetitions.

Do:

◆ Keep your abdominals tight and your back erect.
◆ Keep your head and trunk against the back pad.

Don't be surprised to see people (usually women) doing hundreds of reps of abduction and adduction exercises in the hope of burning fat and *slimming* their thighs. The problem is that when a muscle works hard enough it gets *bigger*, not smaller. (Those guys doing biceps curls all day aren't trying to get their arms to shrink!) Furthermore, the muscle that's exercising has nothing to do with where fat is burned. So although there are reasons to work these muscles, shrinking your thighs isn't one of them.

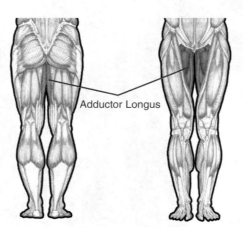
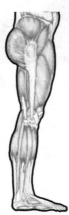
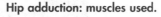

Adductor Longus

Hip adduction: muscles used.

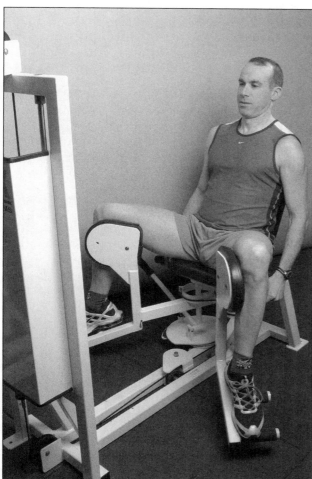

Hip adduction start/finish position.

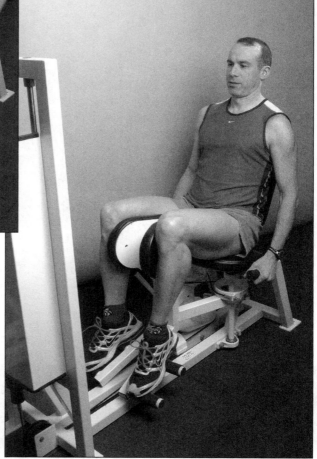

Hip adduction middle position.

In This Chapter

◆ Learning what is deeply felt and rarely seen

◆ Lifting lots with lats

◆ Hoisting away

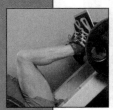 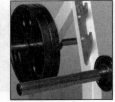 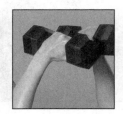 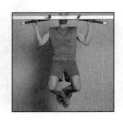 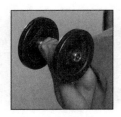 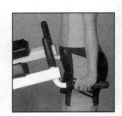

Chapter 8

Flip Side

If you've ever spent any time thinking about your back, as we have, it's rather funny what an overactive (and underused) mind comes up with. Although there's nothing inherently funny about a back, it's a rather odd body part. Here's a large group of muscles that are integral to our strength and well-being, but we rarely get to see it and consequently think about it far less than we do our chest, shoulders, and abdominals.

Latissimus dorsi (or lats) are what gives us that V shape—that rear view bystanders get to admire while we stare straight ahead. The lats are broad muscles that span the area from just behind each armpit to the center of your lower back. These muscles are key for hoisting yourself up while rock climbing, rowing, and performing pull-ups—to name just a few.

For men, large lats provide that wide expanse of muscle that resembles the top of a manta ray. Many women who weight train notice that well-developed lats offer the illusion that their waist is narrower. In fact, it's not; it only appears that way, but few women we know complain about this complimentary illusion.

Just above the lats are the traps or *trapezius* muscles. These powerful muscles run from just below the back of your skull to the edge of your shoulders, and down through the center of your back. When you shrug your shoulders, you're using your traps.

What else is going on in that back of yours? The *rhomboids*—major and minor—span the area between your spine and your shoulder blades. Along with your traps, the rhomboids retract or squeeze your shoulder blades together. The rhomboids are shaped like a Christmas tree and are attached to the innermost part of your shoulder blades (scapula). Any exercise that brings the shoulder blades together works these muscles.

Why Bother?

Aside from looking good, strong back muscles are important for maintaining good posture and vice versa. Meaning: good posture equals a strong healthy back, and a strong back contributes to good posture. Slouching overstretches the muscles, making them work harder during the day. Because overworked muscles fatigue and often spasm, keeping your muscles at their proper working length and strength will prevent this (again, assuming you pay attention to your posture).

Here are three other reasons to train your back:

◆ Strong upper-back muscles enable you to maintain an erect sitting posture without fatigue. Slouching, a bad habit that accounts for untold amounts of chronic back pain, puts these muscles in an overstretched position. This weakens them and leads to muscle spasms, headaches, and backaches.

◆ Strong lats can help you scale that rock wall or give you more power while on the rowing machine, in a swimming pool, or while you paddle a canoe or kayak.

◆ Strong upper-back muscles prevent muscle strength imbalances and protect the shoulders, especially in sports such as swimming, tennis, and pitching, in which emphasis is placed on the anterior shoulders and pectoralis muscles.

The lats, being so large and expansive, respond well to both freeweights and machines. As a matter of fact, you can probably work them much harder with machines than with freeweights, because you're able to use a little more weight and don't have to concentrate on form quite as much as you would with freeweights. However, it is still important to use both, especially when you concentrate on the smaller back muscles such as the rhomboids.

Following are a number of exercises that help develop overall strength, as well as specific back strength.

Deadlifts

One of the three powerlifting exercises, the *deadlift* is one of those good news/bad news deals. First the good news: the deadlift is one of the best overall body exercises you can do. Every muscle is involved during the deadlift— upper back, hips, quads, hamstrings, abdominals— you name it. Now the bad news: it's an advanced lift and must be performed with perfect form or you'll risk injury. We omit it from beginning programs, but it can become a valuable weapon in your back-training arsenal as your strength training progresses.

The most important thing to keep in mind during this lift is that your back must be held as erect as possible. Never allow your chest to go over the bar—this will bring your body forward as you lift the weight, causing you to use your lower back for most of the lift instead of your hips and legs. As you pull the weight, think of pushing your feet through the floor so you really get your legs into it.

Spot Me

When deadlifting with 45-pound plates, the bar begins just below your knees. The problem is that most people must learn the exercise with significantly less weight than that, which lowers the bar and increases how far you need to bend to get the bar. Try starting off using dumbbells instead of a barbell to avoid back strain associated with bending too far.

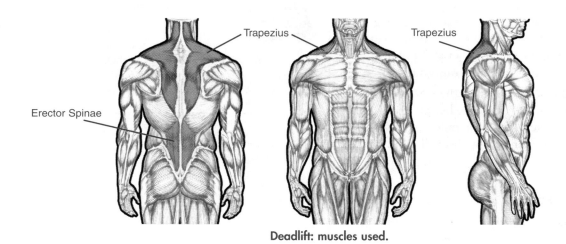

Deadlift: muscles used.

Here is how you properly perform a deadlift:

1. Place your feet slightly wider apart than shoulder width.

2. Reach down and grasp the bar on the outside of the legs with a *reverse grip*.

3. Lower your hips until your thighs are close to parallel to the floor.

4. Flatten your lower back, and look up slightly.

5. Be sure your weight is on your heels, not your toes. Form is of the utmost importance here, so be sure the first time you do this awesome lift you do it with just the bar.

6. Stand upright by straightening your legs and upper body; pause and then slowly return to the initial starting position. Think of yourself as a piston or as an arrow being shot out of the bow.

7. Look up toward the ceiling, because that's where you want to go. (Typically, your body goes where your head and eyes go.) If you look straight ahead, you may come out of the lift going forward. Look up, and you'll usually come out going up.

8. As you lower the bar to the starting position, be sure to keep the bar close to your shins. In fact, the bar should actually graze your shins throughout the lift.

Flex Facts

In the alternating grip or reverse grip, you hold the bar with the fingers of one hand facing your body, and the fingers of your other hand facing away from your body. This improves your ability to hold the bar without it slipping out of your hands.

When performing a deadlift, **don't:**

◆ Lift your hips too quickly. This will transfer most of the effort to your lower back. Your legs, hips, and lower back should be working together, with most of the work done by your legs and hips.

◆ Snap or lock out your knees as you straighten your legs.

◆ Lean back excessively.

◆ Bounce the weight off the floor between repetitions.

Do:

◆ Keep your abdominals tight and your back as erect as possible.

◆ Keep your shoulder blades pulled together—this will help keep your back erect.

Weight a Minute

Don't attempt this exercise if you have lower back problems. People with long torsos often have difficulty performing this lift because the lower back often becomes the pivot point.

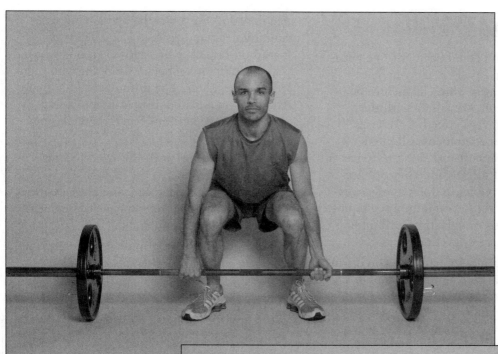

Deadlift start/finish position.

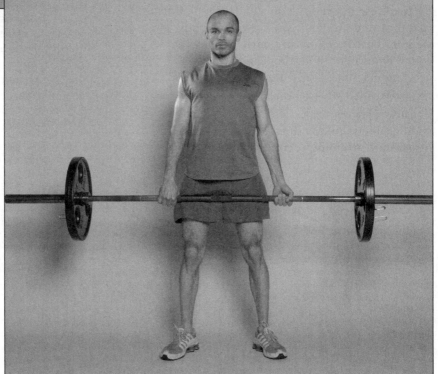

Deadlift middle position.

Pull-Ups and Chin-Ups

If we were in jail and could have just one apparatus, we'd pine for a pull-up/chin-up bar. These simple exercises, which happen to be uncommonly difficult, are (along with the push-up and sit-up) very effective exercises when your access to equipment is limited. Here's the skinny on pull-ups: don't try once or twice and give up. Pull-ups and chin-ups are hard for nearly everyone, so don't get discouraged. If you stick with it, you'll improve rapidly because it's such a thorough strength-building exercise. The keys are effort and focus.

If weak arms and gravity have got you down, try doing an assisted chin-up or pull-up on a machine that allows you to lift only a percentage of your body weight. The *Gravitron* was the first of this type and is still the most popular, but many others can be found in gyms today. To use these machines, you stand on a platform that pushes up to help you hoist your body weight. The directions are fairly simple; the rough equivalent of getting candy out of a vending machine—only much better for you.

Here's how effective this exercise can be. Because a strong back is essential for a kayak paddler, Joe regularly does pull-ups as part of his strength-training regimen. (In fact, most paddlers do.) For years, he and a mate were running neck-and-neck in virtually every marathon race they did. However, one season Joe's paddling mate began whipping him regularly on the water. The difference? His friend had gone on a mad pull-up crusade, doing 20 sets of 10 repetitions regularly while Joe watched late-night TV.

Sound like a lot? It is; however, Joe has another friend who can do 100 consecutive pull-ups. This amazing specimen has a back as wide as a barn door and happens to be one of the best paddlers in Australia.

Adhering to a regular pull-up regimen will have a major impact on your lats.

Bar Talk

The **Gravitron** machine allows users to select either a percentage of their body weight or an amount of plated weight to assist them with the pull-up/chin-up. For example, if you weigh 150 pounds, you can set the machine to give you 50 percent assistance with the exercise, so you'd be pulling or chinning 75 pounds. Or you can select plated weights to give you 70 pounds of assistance.

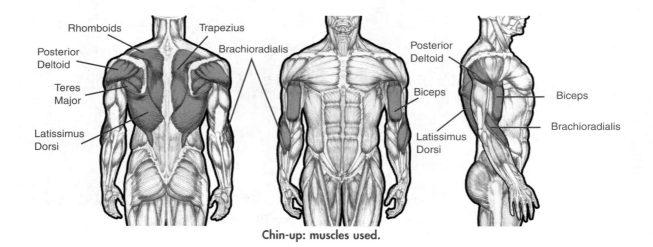

Chin-up: muscles used.

Flex Facts

At age 63, South Korea's Lee Chin-Yong holds the world record with 370 consecutive pull-ups. Not impressed? Robert Chisnail performed a record 22 consecutive one-armed pull-ups on a gymnastics ring!

Here is how you properly perform an assisted chin-up:

1. Grab hold of the chin bar with your hands several inches wider apart than shoulder width.

2. Keep your palms facing toward your body. Lift your feet off the floor, and cross your legs at your ankles.

3. Pull your body to the heavens and touch your upper chest to the bar. (Most people try to inch their chin over the top. By focusing on your chest, you ensure you really work your back.)

4. Pause briefly and return gradually (don't drop down) to the initial starting position with your arms fully extended to get a good stretch.

Spot Me

The difference between the pull-up and the chin-up is the hand position. For pull-ups, palms face away from the body. For chin-ups, palms face toward the body. The underhand grip tends to stress the biceps muscles more, while the overhand emphasizes the muscles of the back more.

Concentrating on your breathing is extremely helpful. Remember on the positive or upward phase to exhale smoothly; reverse on the way down.

When performing an assisted chin-up, **don't**:

◆ Arch your back as you lift your body.

◆ Swing your legs or pull your knees up to help you reach the bar.

◆ Drop from the top position.

Do:

◆ Keep your abdominals tight.

◆ Perform all repetitions in a slow, controlled manner.

◆ Breathe, breathe, breathe.

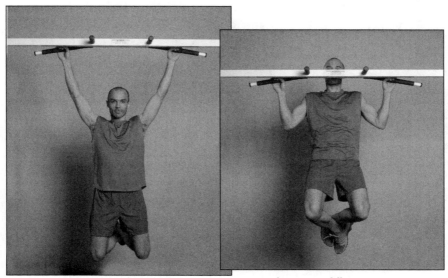

Chin-up start/finish position.   Chin-up middle position.

Row, Row, Row

Dumbbell rows emphasize the lats, middle traps, and rhomboids. The key to performing dumbbell rows is choosing a weight that allows you to squeeze the shoulder blade back on the positive phase of the movement, with control. If you have to jerk the dumbbell up with your body, you're not performing an effective set, meaning your muscles are not getting any stronger, no matter how much weight you're hoisting.

Another key to performing this exercise effectively without causing harm is to keep the leg on the side you're working on the floor. This lends support to your back as you're leaning forward. (Unsupported forward flexion is a major cause of lower back pain.)

With so many back exercises available, must you do this one? It depends on what you feel comfortable with. You certainly don't need to perform every single back exercise there is. The variety is to give you a mental break from doing the same things all the time. Deidre never does dumbbell rows. Why? Because even though her training is as regular as a Swiss watch, she's pretty lazy and would rather work both arms together than one arm at a time (hence she favors cable rows or pull-ups). Once you learn the ropes, you'll see that whether you do this or any of the other exercises is really a matter of personal preference.

Here is how you properly perform a dumbbell row:

1. Place your left hand and your left knee on a bench, and position your right foot on the floor at a comfortable distance from the bench.

2. Reach down with your right hand and grab the dumbbell.

3. Lift the dumbbell off the floor, keeping your right arm straight. Your right palm should be facing the bench.

4. Keeping your upper arm near your torso, slowly pull the dumbbell up to your right shoulder as if you were sawing a piece of wood.

5. Pause briefly, and slowly return the dumbbell to the starting position.

6. Repeat with your left arm (with your right hand and right knee on the bench).

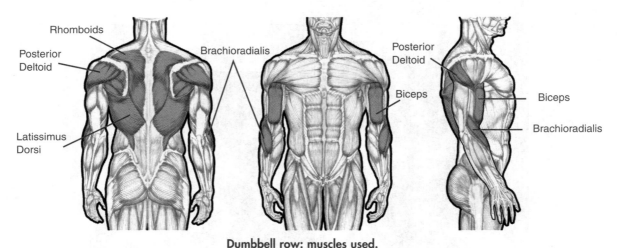

Dumbbell row: muscles used.

When performing a dumbbell row, **don't**:

◆ Arch your back.

◆ Move your shoulder excessively.

◆ Swing your body in an effort to hoist the weight.

◆ Twist your torso.

Do:

◆ Keep your abdominals tight and your back erect.

◆ Keep your shoulder and torso down and parallel to the floor.

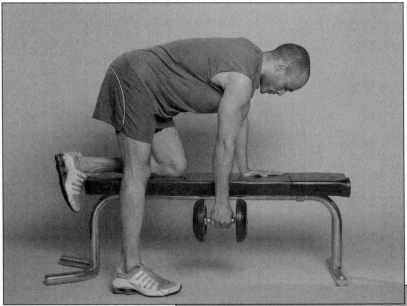

Dumbbell row start/finish position.

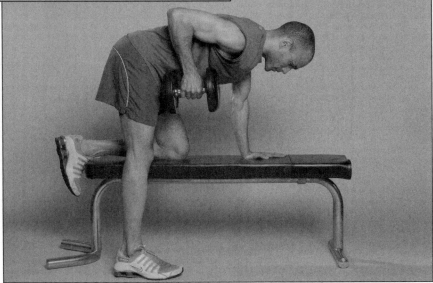

Dumbbell row middle position.

Upright Rows

Many people think of the upright row as a shoulder exercise. In fact, it is a good way to work your deltoids and biceps, but it's a great way to hit the top section of your trapezius, which is why we've included it in the back section.

Here is how you properly perform an upright row:

1. Stand with your feet shoulder-width apart.

2. Hold the barbell slightly less than shoulder-width apart with your palms facing your thighs.

3. Pull the bar up until your hands are about level with your shoulders. Your elbows should be slightly higher than your hands.

4. Pause briefly, and slowly return to the initial starting position.

When performing an upright row, **don't:**

◆ Allow the bar to move away from your body while performing the repetition.

◆ Rock your body back and forth in an effort to lift the weight.

Do:

◆ Keep your abdominals tight and your back erect without leaning backward.

◆ Keep your elbows higher than your hands throughout the range of motion.

Weight a Minute

People with shoulder impingement syndrome (a painful condition in which various structures are compressed in the shoulder joint when the arm is raised) should not perform this exercise.

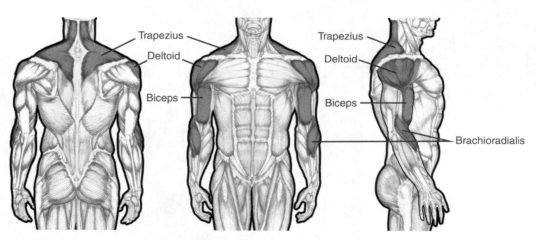

Upright rows: muscles used.

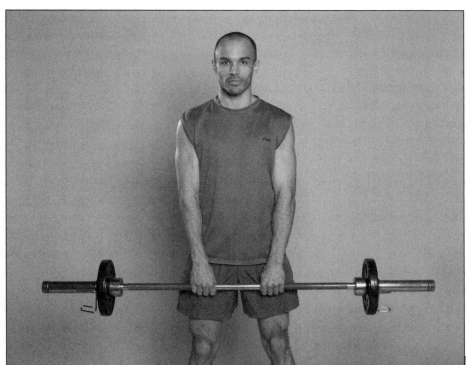

Upright row start/finish position.

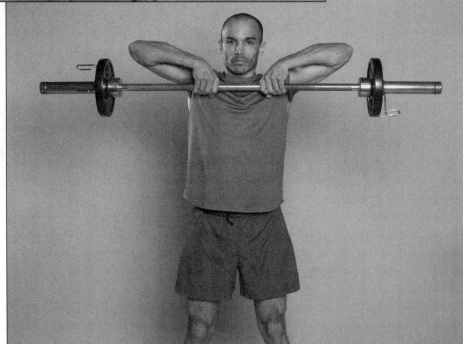

Upright row middle position.

Shrugs

While the upright row works your biceps and deltoids in addition to your trapezius, shrugs work the traps without involving those other muscles. Shrugs may look like a silly, insignificant exercise, but they're a great way to strengthen the traps. (To the uninitiated, someone doing shrugs looks terrifically undecided.) For anyone involved in contact sports or ones in which neck and head injuries are a possibility, the added neck stability shrugs can develop can be crucial.

Here is how you properly perform a shrug:

1. Stand with your feet shoulder-width apart.
2. Hold the dumbbells wider apart than shoulder width with your palms facing your thighs.

3. Keeping your arms and legs straight, move the bar as high as possible by trying to touch your shoulders to your ears.
4. Pause briefly, and slowly return to the initial starting position.

When performing a shrug, **don't**:

◆ Let your range of motion decrease as you get tired.
◆ Rock your body back and forth in an effort to lift the weight.

Do:

◆ Keep your abdominal muscles tight and your back erect without leaning backward.
◆ Perform this exercise with a barbell for a change.

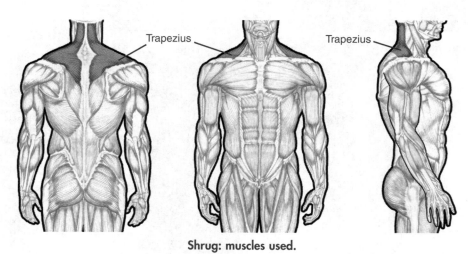

Trapezius   Trapezius

Shrug: muscles used.

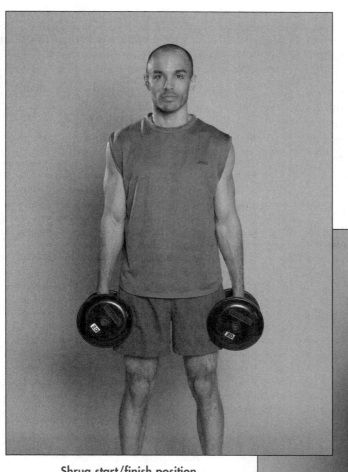

Shrug start/finish position.

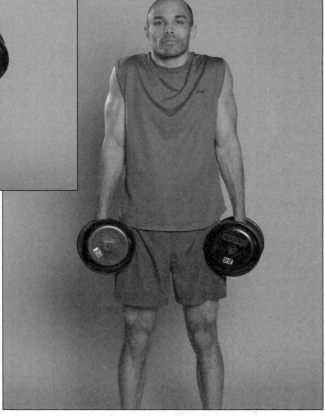

Shrug middle position.

Lat Time

Lat pull-downs are a standard part of virtually every lifter's routine. Done correctly, a lat pull-down will turn a blocky or narrow back into that much-sought-after V shape. Furthermore, if you're a swimmer, rock climber, rower, or any type of athlete who would benefit from a powerful upper body, this exercise is for you.

There are two types of lat pull-downs: behind the neck or to the chest. With the behind-the-neck exercise, you might have a tendency to jut your neck forward, putting it in an awkward position, especially if you're using too much weight. For this reason, we prefer the chest variation because the neck is kept in a more stable position.

Here is how you properly perform a lat pull-down:

1. Grab the bar with your palms facing away from your body, slightly wider apart than shoulder width.
2. Sit on the seat with your knees under the pads. (Remember to adjust the pads if your knees don't fit snuggly, yet comfortably.)
3. Lean back slightly.
4. Pull the bar to your collarbone.
5. Pause briefly, and slowly return to the initial starting position.

When performing a lat pull-down, **don't**:

◆ Come out of your seat on the way up.
◆ Swing your body back and forth in an effort to lift the weight.
◆ Slouch as you bring the weight down.

Do:

◆ Keep your abs tight and your back erect.
◆ Squeeze your shoulder blades together as you bring the weight down behind your neck.
◆ Control the weight throughout the range of motion.

Weight a Minute

Lat pull-downs are contraindicated for those with shoulder impingement syndrome, because the exercise can aggravate the condition.

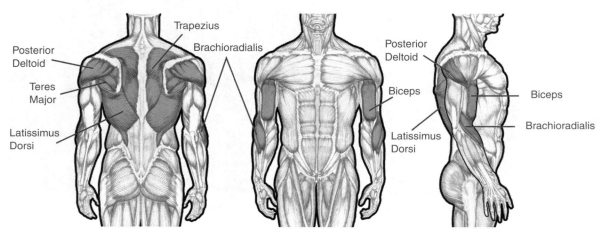

Lat pull-down: muscles used.

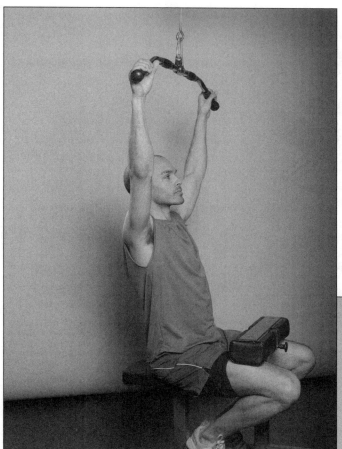

Lat pull-down start/finish position.

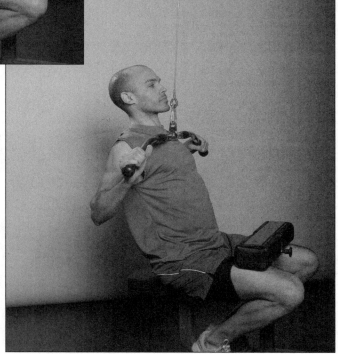

Lat pull-down middle position.

Cable Rows

The cable-row machine works the lats, middle traps, and rhomboids. You should remember to keep your back erect even as you lean forward to return to the start position. As you pull the handle toward you—the initial pull is where your lats are worked—remember to keep your chest up and squeeze your shoulder blades together. (This is where the traps and rhomboids are worked.) Like virtually every exercise we recommend, cable rows should be performed slowly, with the exhalation coming on the positive phase of the movement (in this case, the pull toward the chest).

Spot Me

Several different handles are available for this exercise. Experiment with them until you decide which one feels the most comfortable.

Here is how you properly perform a cable row:

1. Sit down, and place your feet against the foot platform.
2. Grab the bar, and lean back slightly.
3. Pull the bar to your midsection.
4. Pause briefly, and slowly return to the starting position with your arms fully extended.

When performing a cable row, **don't**:

◆ Swing your upper body back and forth in an effort to lift the weight.
◆ Allow the weight stack being lifted to slam or bounce against the remainder of the weight stack between repetitions.
◆ Perform the exercise rapidly.
◆ Arch your back.

Do:

◆ Keep your abdominals tight and your back erect.
◆ Keep your knees slightly bent.
◆ Squeeze your shoulder blades together at the finish position.

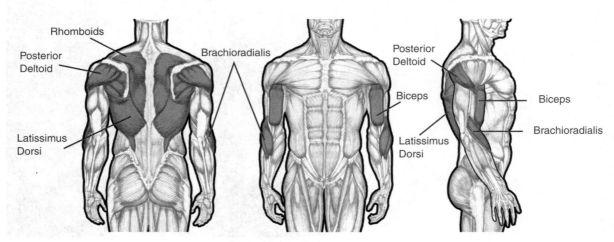

Cable rows: muscles used.

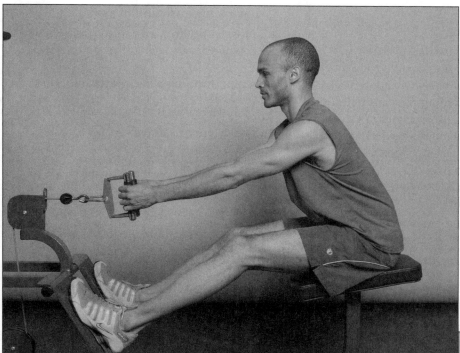

Cable row
start/finish position.

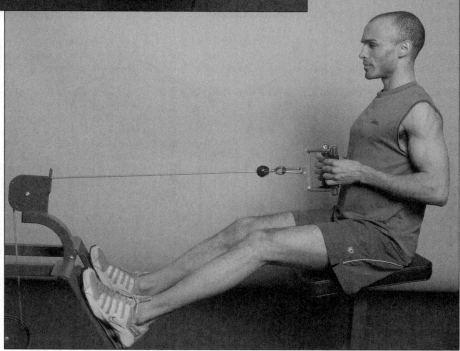

Cable row middle position.

Extension

Most of the exercises in this chapter focus on the muscles of your upper and middle back, but we've yet to get to the *erector spinae* muscles of your lower back. Strengthening those muscles is crucial in ensuring proper posture and in the prevention of lower back pain. Considering that the majority of people experience lower back pain at some time in their lives, it's not a bad idea to do whatever's possible to decrease your chances of being a statistic.

The 45° back extension bench is an effective and safe way to work those erector spinae.

Here is how you properly perform a back extension:

1. Be sure your heels are securely placed behind the foot platform.
2. Begin by "folding" at the waist and letting your head hang down toward the floor.
3. Raise your torso until it's straight.
4. Pause at the fully extended position, and slowly return to the starting position.

When performing a back extension, **don't**:

◆ Push with your legs.
◆ Throw your head back.
◆ Swing back quickly.
◆ Hyperextend your back or neck.

Do:

◆ Keep your head in a neutral position.
◆ Control your weight in both directions.

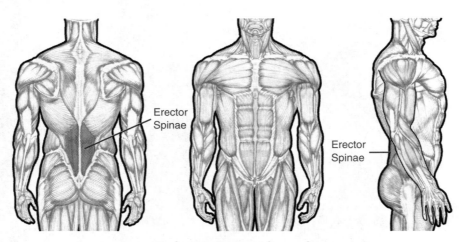

Erector Spinae

Erector Spinae

Back extension: muscles used.

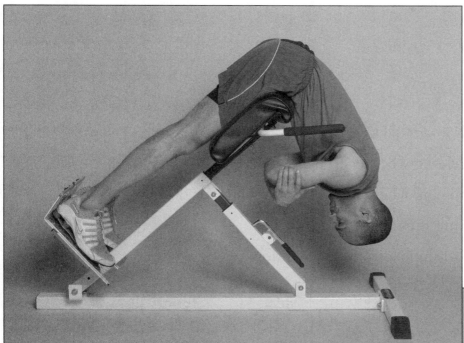

**Back extension
start/finish position.**

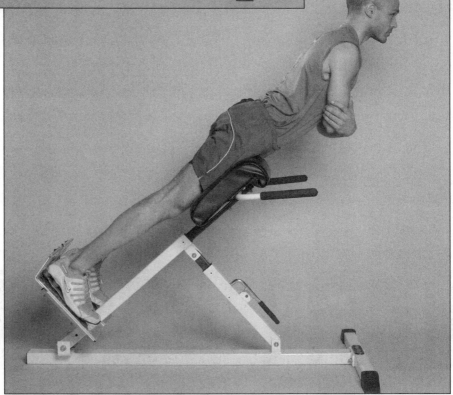

Back extension middle position.

In This Chapter

- ◆ Deciding whether to bench or bust
- ◆ Knowing whether to go flat, incline, or decline
- ◆ Doing dips
- ◆ Learning chest machine options

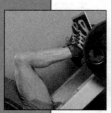 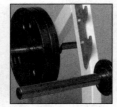 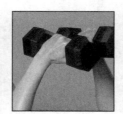 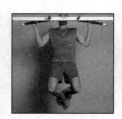 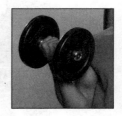 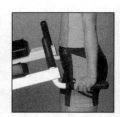

Chapter 9

Chest or Bust

Bulging arms and a chiseled chest may be the ideal for American men, but the bench press—one of the three powerlifting disciplines—is generally the signature lift men use to demonstrate how strong they are. Often you'll hear weight lifters ask each other, "What's your bench?" the way runners ask each other how fast they can run a 10K.

Oddly enough, the bench press, the exercise that builds the muscles in your chest, may be the most abused and overpopularized lift of them all. Why? A thick, sculpted chest is the body part men often assume will impress women. Because this lift has become such a *benchmark* of strength, too many men put too much weight on the bar too much of the time. The result often leads to shoulder injuries as well as bruised egos.

Pecs to Flex

The *pectoral* muscles (pecs) span the upper chest wall and are largely responsible for pushing and throwing movements. There are actually two pectoral muscles—the *pectoralis major* (the muscle we're concentrating on for weight-lifting purposes) and the *pectoralis minor*, which depresses the scapula (or shoulder blade); the pectoralis minor often gets extremely tight in people who have poor posture and needs to be massaged to get released.

Why strong pecs? Because of the following reasons:

◆ If you play baseball or any other sport involving throwing, strong pecs can give you that added *oomph*.

◆ If you're a swimmer, building your pecs will get you from one side of the pool to the other a bit quicker.

◆ If you're taking boxing classes or practicing the martial arts, strong pecs can make your punch a little harder.

Following are some basic exercises to get you started in the gym. Remember …

◆ Do them all slowly and under control—your muscles and joints will thank you.

◆ Breathe out as you push; breathe in as you return to the starting position.

The Bench

The bench press, also known as the chest press, is a standard part of virtually every strength program. Its primary focus is on the pectoralis major muscles, although it also works the front of the deltoid and the triceps. As we mentioned earlier, don't get caught up in the "How much can you lift?" game. Focus on form, and the strength gains will take care of themselves.

Here is how you properly perform a bench press:

1. Lie on your back with your feet either flat on the floor or, if your feet don't touch the floor, without your back arching.

2. Bend your knees, and put your feet on the bench. (When you put your feet on the bench, you reduce the potential stress on your back and isolate the muscles a bit more. It also means you'll use less weight.) In either case, keep your back flat.

3. Grab the bar with a grip slightly wider apart than shoulder width.

4. Lift the bar from the uprights, or have a spotter assist you.

5. Slowly lower the bar to your chest, stopping at the highest part of your chest (at the nipple line); then return to the initial starting position.

Weight a Minute

The temptation to try a maximal lift on a bench press (or any other lift) is one we urge you to ignore. One-rep maximal lifts place an enormous orthopedic stress on your body and tend to shoot your blood pressure through the roof. Leave maximal lifts to competitive lifters.

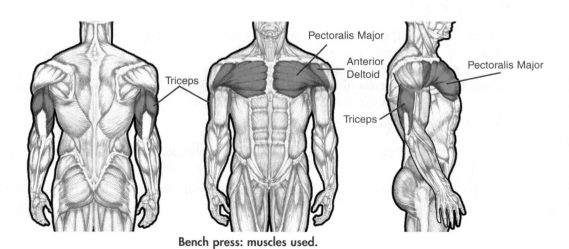

Bench press: muscles used.

When performing a bench press, **don't**:

◆ Arch your back.

◆ Lift your buttocks off the bench.

◆ Move your legs or feet—keep them stationary for better support.

◆ Snap or lock out your elbows at the end position.

◆ Bounce the barbell off your chest.

◆ Hold your breath.

Do:

◆ Keep your abdomen tight and back flat.

◆ Use a firm but relaxed grip.

Flex Facts

The bench press is significantly different for powerlifters than for noncompetitive athletes. In competition, powerlifters arch their backs, dig their feet into the floor, and grind their shoulder blades into the bench. This anchoring gives them enough leverage to drive the bar up off their chest to successfully make their one repetition max.

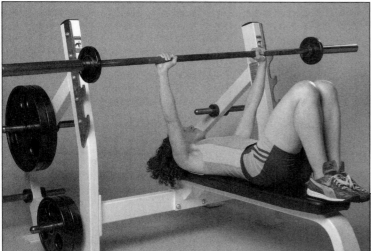

Bench press start/finish position.

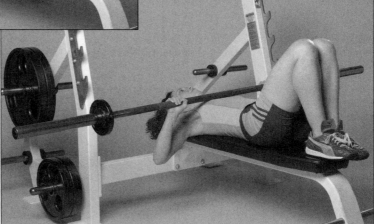

Bench press middle position.

Goin' Uphill

The incline bench press works on the upper part of your pecs. Bodybuilders tend to focus on defining every single muscle possible so they will perform flat, incline, and decline bench presses to bring out their pecs as much as they can.

Here is how you properly perform an incline press:

1. Lie on the bench, and place your feet either flat on the floor or on the footrest (if one is present).
2. Grab the bar with a grip slightly wider apart than shoulder width.
3. Lift the bar from the uprights, or have a spotter assist you.
4. Slowly lower the bar until it touches the upper part of your chest, just below your collarbone; then slowly return to the initial starting position.

When performing an incline press, **don't**:

◆ Lift your buttocks off the bench.
◆ Arch your back.
◆ Move your legs or your feet.
◆ Bounce the barbell off your chest.
◆ Snap or lock out your elbows at the end range.
◆ Hold your breath.

Do:

◆ Keep your abdomen tight and your back flat.
◆ Be sure to lower the bar to just below your collarbone.

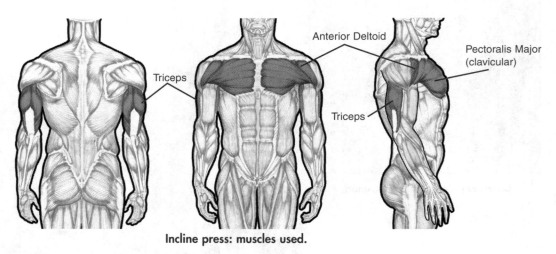

Incline press: muscles used.

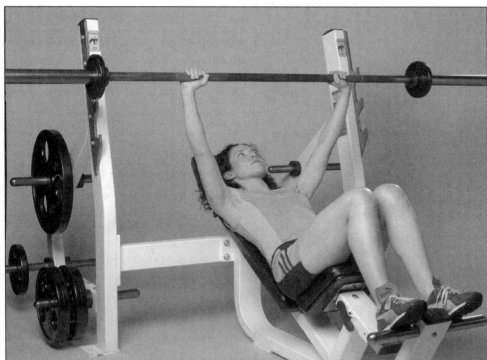

Incline press
start/finish position.

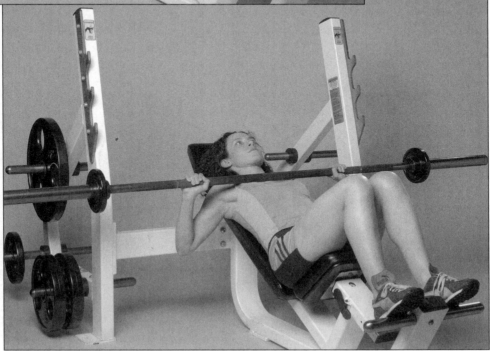

Incline press middle position.

Down We Go

The decline bench is the kissin' cousin of the incline variety because it works the lower part of your chest. Essentially, you follow the same procedure as the flat and incline bench. The tricky part is sliding under the bar without smacking your head.

Here is how you properly perform a decline press:

1. Lie down on the bench, putting your feet under the support provided.

2. Grab the bar with a grip slightly wider apart than shoulder width.

3. Lift from the uprights, or have a spotter assist you.

4. Slowly lower the bar to your chest just below the nipple line; then return to the initial starting position.

When performing a decline press, **don't**:

◆ Lock your elbows out as you straighten your arms.

◆ Bounce the bar off your chest.

◆ Arch your back.

◆ Hold the bar with a suicide grip!

Weight a Minute

The suicide grip (or thumbless grip) refers to gripping the barbell with your thumb on the same side of the barbell as your four other fingers. Some lifters find this more comfortable, but it is extremely dangerous because there is the possibility the bar will slip from your hands. We don't recommend it.

Do:

◆ Keep your abdominals tight.

◆ Keep your head on the bench.

◆ Lower the bar to your nipple line.

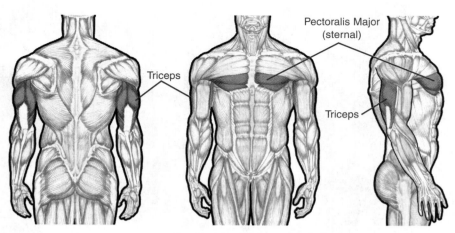

Triceps

Pectoralis Major (sternal)

Triceps

Decline press: muscles used.

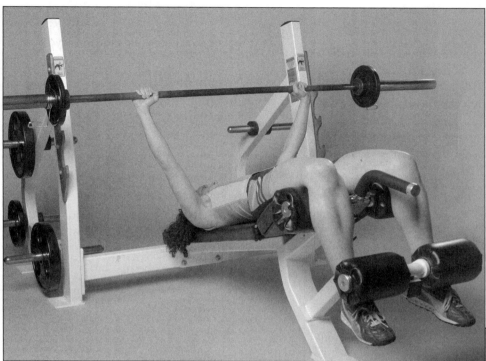

**Decline press
start/finish position.**

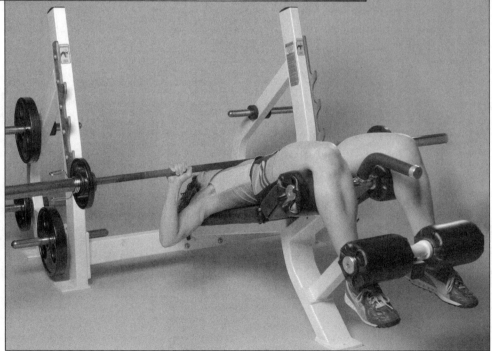

Decline press middle position.

Dips

Most people find dips extremely difficult, with good reason—they are. They also happen to be one of the best exercises for your chest and upper body that money can buy. If you can't do even one, don't despair. Nowadays, most well-equipped gyms have an assisted dip machine or Gravitron that help you by pushing up as you stand on a platform. Better to use the help than to use bad form with your full body weight.

Here is how you properly perform a dip:

1. Stand between the two handles, bend your knees, and hold yourself up by keeping your elbows straight. If you're using an assisted dip machine, keep your feet flat on the platform.

2. Slowly bend your elbows, lowering your body as far as you can comfortably—ideally, until your upper arms are parallel to the floor; then return to the initial starting position with a smooth, outward breath.

When performing a dip, **don't:**

◆ Snap or lock out your elbows as you push yourself up.

◆ Arch your back.

◆ Allow your elbows to jut out toward the side; keep them pointed directly backward.

Do:

◆ Keep your chest up.

◆ Keep your chin tucked and your eyes focused on an object directly in front of you.

◆ Keep your knees bent.

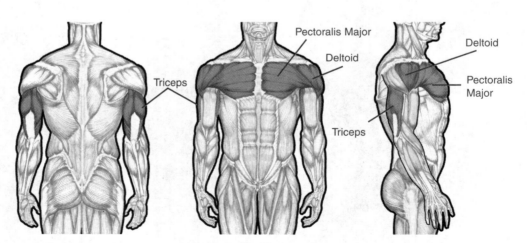

Dips: muscles used.

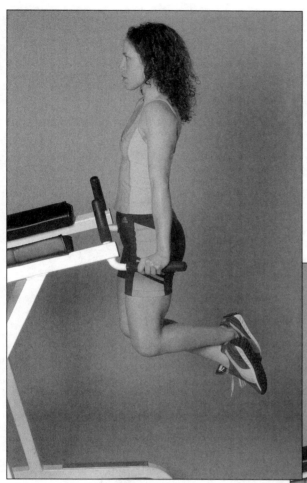

Dip start/finish position.

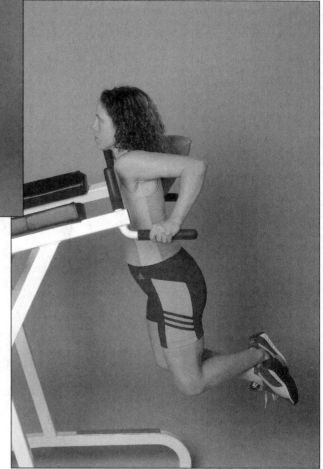

Dip middle position.

Push, Please

The push-up is perhaps the most classic of all strength-training exercises. Think back to grade school when you did that first facsimile of what Marines and Navy SEALs do more of than any other exercise. While the push-up is as common as a pigeon in New York City, it is an important exercise to incorporate into your regimen, especially considering the fact that you can do it anywhere, at any time.

Here is how you properly perform a push-up:

1. Lie on the floor with your legs together and your hands on the floor pointing forward and just outside your shoulders.

2. Keep your back and legs straight.

3. Slowly push your body from the floor until your elbows are straight, then slowly return to the initial starting position. Concentrate on keeping your back straight and your rhythm even.

When performing a push-up, **don't**:

◆ Allow your back to sag while assuming the up position.

◆ Snap or lock out your elbows while at the end position.

◆ Rest in between the start position and the end position.

Do:

◆ Keep your abdomen tight.

◆ Keep your head facing the floor without arching your neck.

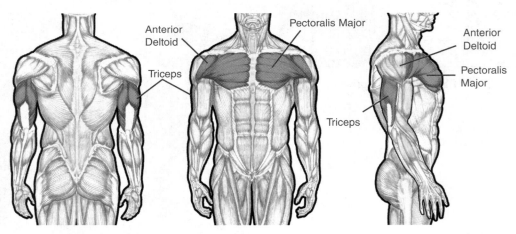

Push-ups: muscles used.

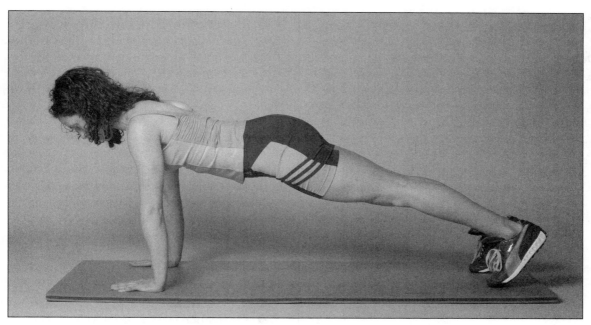

Push-up start/finish position.

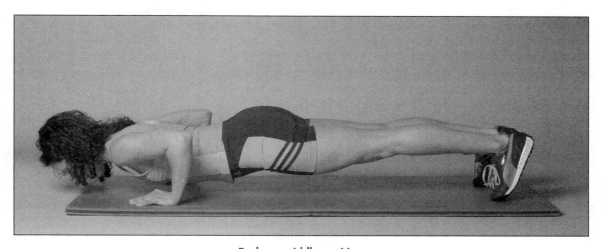

Push-up middle position.

Flying Solo

Dumbbell flyes are an extremely challenging exercise for your chest because they emphasize the pec major without assistance from the anterior delts and the triceps. It's important to concentrate on your form and keep a smooth and continuous flow to this exercise. Any herky-jerkiness is likely to result in injury. If you find yourself cheating, use less weight.

Here is how you properly perform a chest flye:

1. Lie down on the bench with your feet either flat on the floor or your knees bent and your feet on the bench.
2. Stretch out your arms, with one dumbbell in each hand.
3. Slightly bend your elbows.
4. Slowly bring your arms together until the dumbbells almost touch; then return to the initial starting position. Picture the wings of a soaring bird, and you've got the right idea.

When performing a chest flye, **don't:**

◆ Use too much weight with this exercise. You can cause serious injury to your *rotator cuff* muscles in your shoulder.
◆ Straighten your elbows—you can put excessive stress on the joint.
◆ Arch your back.

Do:

◆ Get a good stretch at the start position.
◆ Focus on form.

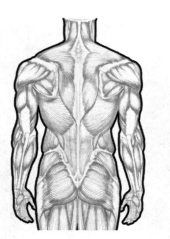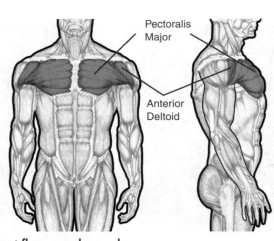

Chest flyes: muscles used.

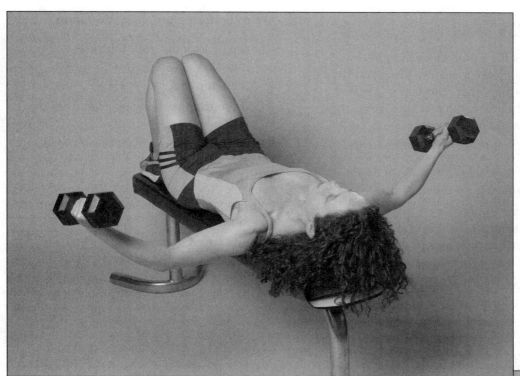

Chest flye start/finish
position.

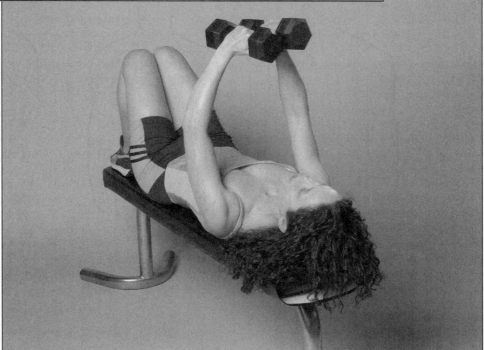

Chest flye middle position.

Chest Press

This machine is the rough equivalent of the flat bench press. Some machines place you flat on your back, while others put you in a seated position. In either case, the machine works the same muscles as the bench press.

Here is how you properly perform a chest press:

1. Position yourself on the machine.
2. Your feet should be flat on the floor or on the footrest, if there is one to use. Remember: posture counts.
3. Place your hands on the handles.
4. Push the handles forward, focusing your attention on your pecs.
5. Finish the forward push just short of full extension; then slowly return to the starting position without relaxing completely.

When performing a chest press, **don't:**

◆ Snap or lock out your elbow as you press forward.
◆ Arch your back.
◆ Lift your upper body or head from the back pad.
◆ Lift your buttocks from the seat pad.

Do:

◆ Keep your feet flat on the floor or on the footrest.
◆ Keep your abdomen tight.

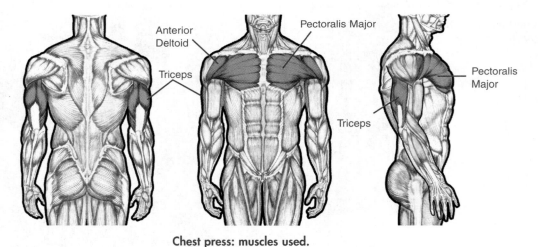

Chest press: muscles used.

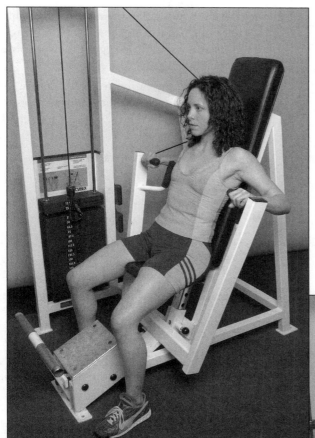

Chest press start/finish position.

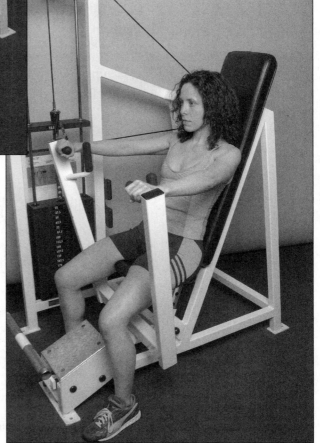

Chest press middle position.

Pec Deck

The pec deck is a terrific machine for isolating the pec muscles. It's analogous to the dumbbell flyes and enables you to isolate your pecs without using the muscles in your arms.

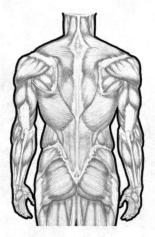

Spot Me _____

The pec deck is the machine version of the flye, but we actually prefer it. Both exercises isolate your pecs and eliminate your arm muscles, but the pec deck enables you to work through a broader range of motion and keeps constant pressure on the muscle.

Here is how you properly perform a pec deck:

1. Position yourself on the machine.
2. Your feet should be flat on the floor or on the footrest.
3. Place your forearms on either side of the pads.

4. Without moving your upper body or lifting your head from the back pad, bring your elbows as close together as possible by pushing against the arm pads.
5. Resist the temptation to twist, squirm, or otherwise recruit any other body parts. Remember that the focus is on form and elegance.
6. Return to the initial starting position.

When performing a pec dec, **don't**:

◆ Lift your elbows off the arm pads.
◆ Lift your upper body or head from the back pad.
◆ Lift your buttocks from the seat pad.
◆ Slam the stack weights between repetitions.
◆ Arch your back.

Do:

◆ Keep your feet flat on the floor or on the footrest.
◆ Keep your abdomen tight.

If you have a shoulder impingement, refrain from doing this exercise.

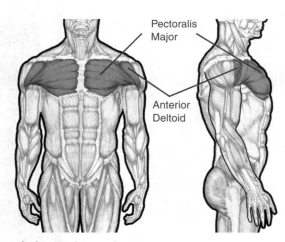

Pec deck: muscles used.

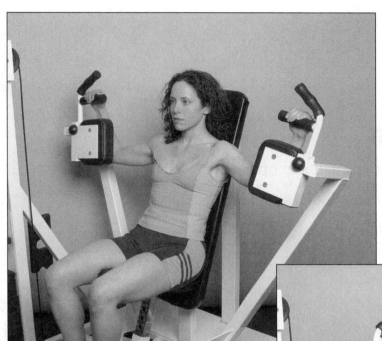

Pec deck start/finish position.

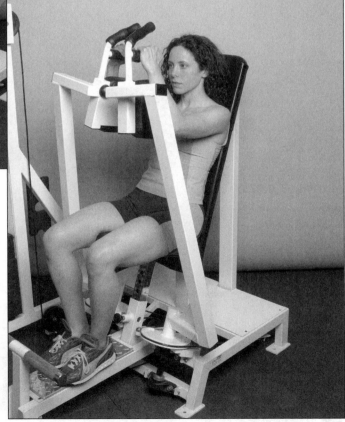

Pec deck middle position.

In This Chapter

- ◆ Remembering the small and oft-neglected shoulders
- ◆ Learning the anatomy of a shoulder
- ◆ Performing delt exercises

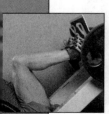
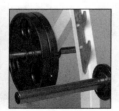
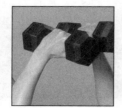
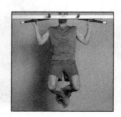
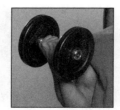
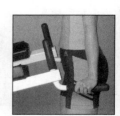

Chapter 10

The World on Your Shoulders

Atlas carried the world on his shoulders. Often you hear people say, "That must be a load off your shoulders!" Or "You've been shouldering a huge burden the last few weeks." In other words, the shoulders are known to bear the brunt of hard work and mental stress. While most people relish training their chest, arms, back, and even their legs, the shoulders are one of the most neglected body parts.

Why? The shoulders (the *deltoids* or delts) are the muscles located at the top of your arm. There are actually three parts to this muscle: the *anterior deltoid*, which raises the arm upward from the front; the *medial deltoid*, which raises the arm upward from the side; and the *posterior deltoid*, which draws the arm backward. Together, these muscles form a triangle on your shoulder (hence the name deltoid—as in the Greek *delta*). These muscles are amazingly versatile but are relatively small and, therefore, fatigue easily. When you start training your shoulders, you're likely to notice, first, how weak they are, and second, how quickly they respond if you train them diligently.

Bar Talk

The **deltoid** is divided into three sections—the **anterior deltoid** is the front section, the **medial deltoid** is in the middle, and the **posterior deltoid** is at the back.

There's another seldom-considered set of muscles that play a large role in the health and welfare of your shoulders you should know about: the rotator cuff. The rotator cuff muscles are located beneath the deltoids, and their function is to keep your long arm bone (the *humerus*) from slipping out of joint. Compared to the deltoids, these muscles are small and seldom thought about—until an injury occurs, often while straining under the load of too much weight on the bench press.

Not sure how your rotator cuff functions? Try this: stick your arm out to the side with your elbow locked. Now twist your arm from side to side. The muscles that get the job done? The loyal rotator cuff. The supraspinatus also assists your deltoids in initiating the outward movement of your arm from the side. And it provides stability to the joint when you throw a ball, Frisbee, javelin—you get the picture. Having said all that, it should come as no surprise to hear that a thorough shoulder workout encompasses the deltoids and the rotator cuff muscles as well.

Flex Facts

Anatomy students always remember the muscles of the rotator cuff with the acronym SITS. The rotator cuff consists of four muscles—supraspinatus, infraspinatus, teres minor, and subscapularis.

Should I?

Why strong shoulders? If you play racquet sports, baseball, or want to be the next Joe Montana, improving your shoulder strength is a must. From a cosmetic point of view, powerfully built shoulders will give your upper body more width. Add buff shoulders to a sculpted back, and your waist will look significantly smaller. (And women take notice: train your shoulders long enough, and you won't need to use those shoulder pads in your clothes.)

It is extremely important to lay down a good foundation when you begin to work on your deltoids. The last thing you need to worry about is the amount of weight you're using. Always be sure your form is excellent and you're not using your whole body to initiate the exercise.

When working your shoulders, it's important to maintain good form and posture and move the weight in a smooth, controlled manner.

Military Action

The military press is a great basic compound exercise to do. It works not only the deltoids but the triceps as well and can be done in both sitting and standing positions. Deidre prefers to perform it while standing because it's easier to control the position of the lower back, especially with heavier weights. No matter which position you choose, keep your back erect, your abdominals tight, and your head in neutral position. If it sounds like we're sticklers for form, that's because we are.

Here is how you properly perform a military press:

1. Sit with your feet on the foot platform, if there is one, with a dumbbell in each hand.
2. Bring the dumbbells up with your palms facing forward.
3. Hold them like a driver signaling to make a right-hand turn—in a position of 90° of shoulder abduction and 90° of elbow flexion.

4. Slowly straighten your arms overhead—finishing with a slight bend in your elbows.
5. While maintaining control of the weight, return to the initial starting position.

When performing a military press, **don't**:

◆ Arch your back.
◆ Clang the dumbbells together.
◆ Allow your elbows to dip below the start position.
◆ Twist from your waist to nudge the weight upward.

Do:

◆ Keep your abs tight.
◆ Keep your head and neck straight.
◆ Pay strict attention to your form.

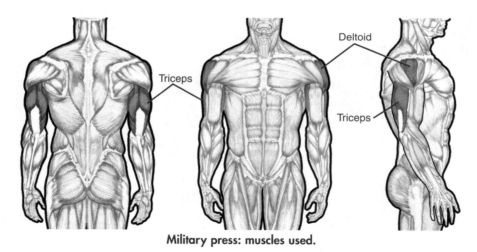

Triceps

Deltoid

Triceps

Military press: muscles used.

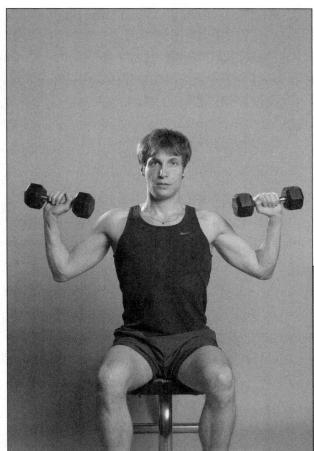

Military press start/finish position.

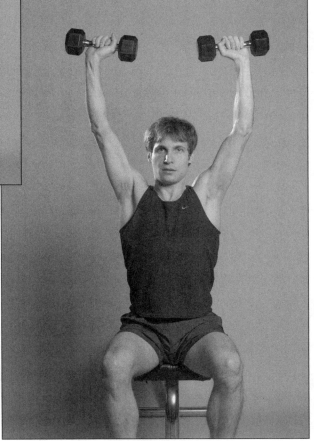

Military press middle position.

Literally Lateral

Lateral raises are a great exercise for isolating the middle deltoids. (They are considered one-joint exercises because the only joint flexing and extending is the shoulder joint. Military presses are two-joint exercises because two joints flex and extend.) Note that you will be using much lighter weight with lateral raises than with the military press. Also note that you'll need to keep your elbows slightly bent to take excess pressure off of them.

Here is how you properly perform a lateral raise:

1. Sit at the end of a bench with your legs together.
2. Hold a dumbbell in each hand at your side with your palms facing your legs.
3. With a slight bend in your elbows, raise the dumbbells away from the sides of your body until your arms are parallel to the floor.
4. Return to the starting position under control.

When performing a lateral raise, **don't:**

◆ Raise your arms much above the parallel position.
◆ Dip your body downward as you lift the weights up.
◆ Lean forward.
◆ Relax completely between repetitions.

Do:

◆ Keep your abdominals tight.
◆ Keep your weight evenly distributed on your feet.
◆ Maintain good posture.

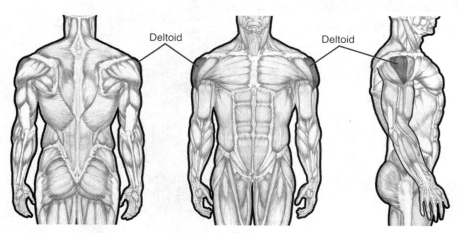

Lateral raise: muscles used.

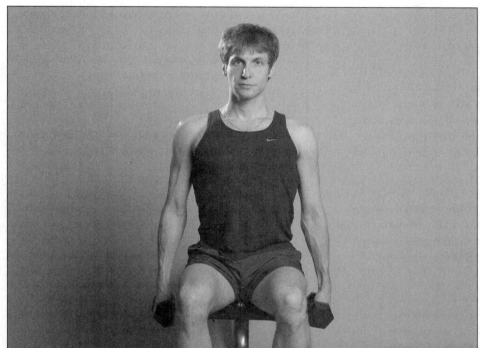

Lateral raise
start/finish position.

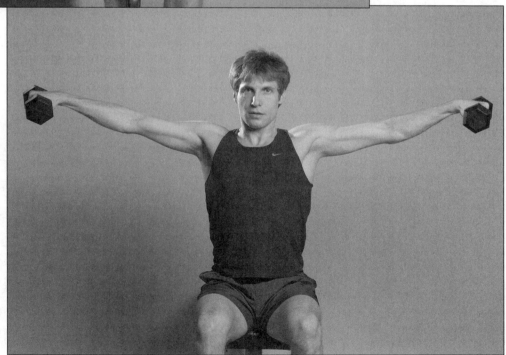

Lateral raise middle position.

Front Raises

If you're wondering why we're listing so many exercises for the shoulder, keep in mind that it is a three-part muscle and that each muscle must be worked to get stronger as a whole. Front raises are another one-joint exercise, meaning they isolate the anterior deltoid, which is the muscle you use to reach up to grab an apple off a tree.

Although you will see people exercise both arms at the same time, we prefer you don't. Doing both at the same time will make it easier for you to cheat by dipping your body down as your raise both your arms up.

Spot Me

Although we have shown the front raise exercise with palms facing downward, people who have shoulder impingement syndrome should not perform it in this fashion because it can worsen the condition. Instead, begin with your palms facing inward, and keep them facing inward throughout the exercise.

Here is how you properly perform a front raise:

1. Stand with your feet shoulder-width apart and your knees slightly bent.
2. Hold a dumbbell in each hand at your sides with your palms facing your legs.
3. Slowly raise one dumbbell up in front of your body until your arm is parallel to the floor.
4. Slowly return to the starting position.
5. Do a complete set with one arm before beginning the next arm.

When performing a front raise, **don't:**

◆ Rock your body back and forth.
◆ Raise your arms above the parallel position.

Do:

◆ Keep your abs tight.
◆ Maintain good posture.

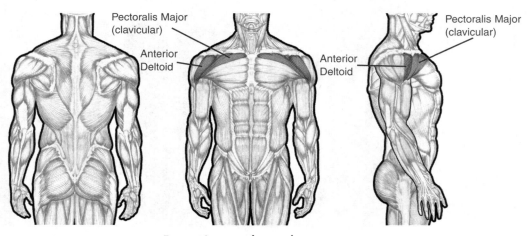

Front raise: muscles used.

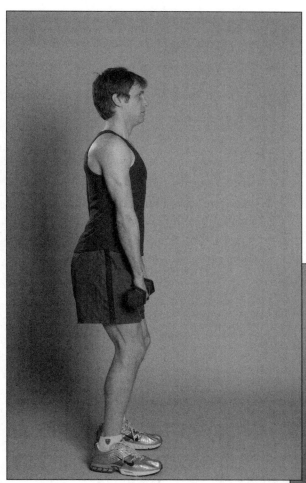

Front raise start/finish position.

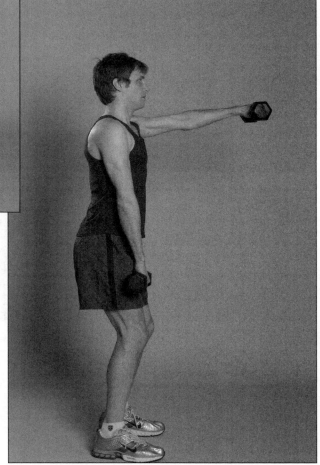

Front raise middle position.

Reverse Flyes

Reverse flyes are another one-joint exercise that isolates the posterior deltoid. For the whole muscle to get strong, all of its parts must be worked.

Here is how you properly perform a reverse flye:

1. Sit on a flat bench, and bend forward at your waist.
2. Let the dumbbells hang down at your sides.
3. With a dumbbell in each hand, bring the dumbbells together, palms facing in.
4. Bend your elbows slightly as you raise the dumbbells away from your body.
5. Focus on squeezing your shoulder blades together.
6. With control, return to the starting position.

When performing a reverse flye, **don't**:

◆ Turn your head left or right.
◆ Raise your arms quickly, forcing your body forward.
◆ Allow the dumbbells to clang as you bring them together.

Do:

◆ Keep your abs tight.
◆ Maintain slow, controlled movement throughout the exercise.
◆ Squeeze your shoulder blades together at the top of the movement.

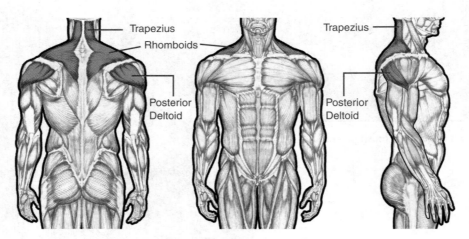

Reverse flyes: muscles used.

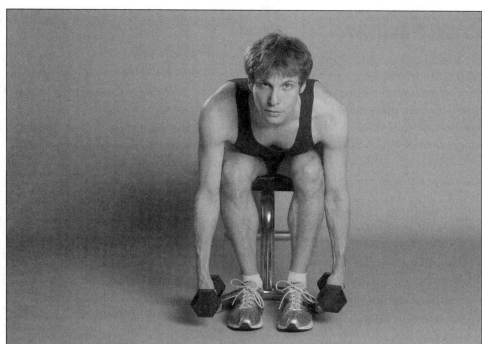

Reverse flye
start/finish
position.

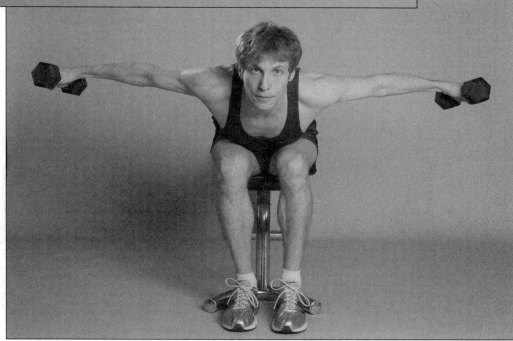

Reverse flye middle position.

Shoulder Press Machine

This machine is the kissin' cousin of the military press; however, unlike the freeweight version, which requires copious amounts of concentration, using the shoulder press machine is safer (and easier) because you neither have to stabilize the weight nor worry about it falling against your will.

Here is how you properly perform a shoulder press:

1. Sit on the bench with your feet shoulder-width apart.
2. Grasp the handles slightly wider than shoulder-width apart.
3. Sit up straight, and start your engine.
4. Push the handles up until your arms are just short of full extension.
5. Return to a position just short of the initial starting position to keep tension on your muscles. Remember to maintain control of the downward part of the lift.

When performing a shoulder press, **don't**:

◆ Lean backward.
◆ Lift your buttocks off the bench.
◆ Allow your elbows to snap or lock in the middle position.
◆ Allow the weight stack being lifted to slam against the remaining weight stack between repetitions.

Do:

◆ Keep your abdominals tight and your back erect.
◆ Keep your head on the bench.

Weight a Minute

People with lower back pain or shoulder impingement syndrome should not do this exercise.

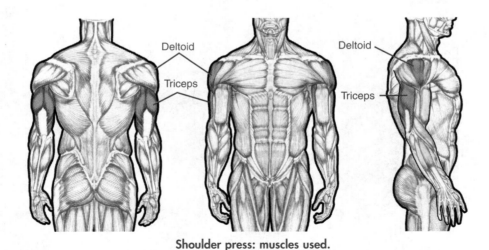

Shoulder press: muscles used.

Deltoid

Triceps

Deltoid

Triceps

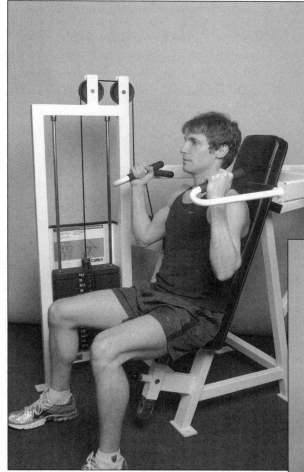

Shoulder press machine start/finish position.

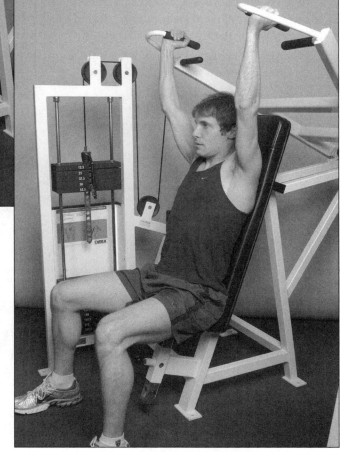

Shoulder press machine middle position.

Lateral Raise Machine

This machine virtually duplicates the freeweight version of the side lateral raise. Some people prefer using a machine because it requires less concentration; others like using freeweights because it may be more comfortable for them and they maintain a bit more control. Try both, and you can make the call.

Here is how you properly perform a lateral raise:

1. Sit on the seat.
2. Position your upper arms against the arm pads, and lay your upper body against the back pad. Your arms should extend straight down, and your elbows should be bent to 90° with your palms facing in.
3. Keep your arms fairly straight, and raise them away from your body until they are parallel to the floor.
4. Return the weight gradually to a position just short of the initial starting position.

When performing a lateral raise, **don't:**

◆ Lift your arms to a position higher than parallel.
◆ Allow the weight stack being lifted to slam against the remaining weight stack between repetitions.

Do:

◆ Keep your upper body and head against the back pad to reduce the strain on your neck and back.
◆ Keep your abdominals tight and your back erect.

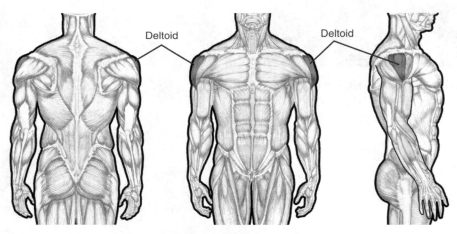

Deltoid   Deltoid

Lateral raise: muscles used.

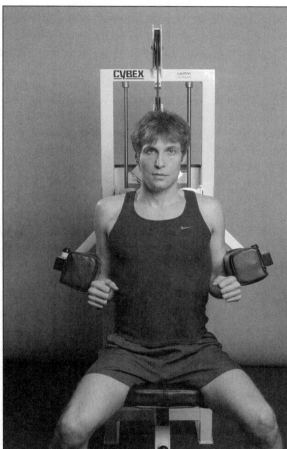

Lateral raise machine start/finish position.

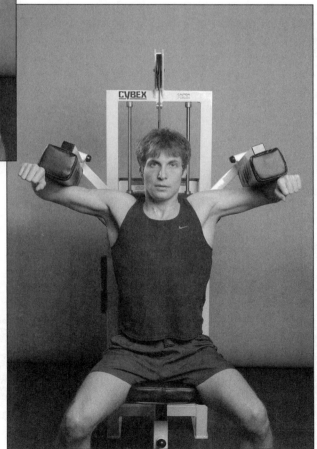

Lateral raise machine middle position.

In This Chapter

- ◆ Bulging biceps turn heads
- ◆ Building your biceps
- ◆ Boosting your triceps

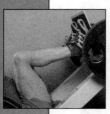 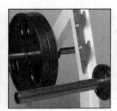 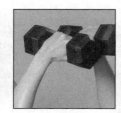 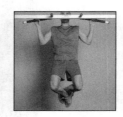 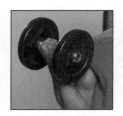 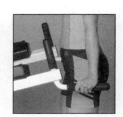

Chapter 11

Armed but Not Dangerous

Picture this: you walk into a gym for your first workout, and you're looking for a trainer. You see two trainers discussing amino acids by the office. Both have pleasing physiques, but one has huge arms. Which one do you want for your trainer? (Be honest.) Our practical experience says you go with Bobby Biceps.

Chew on this amusing "looks can be deceiving" tale: Jonathan used to work with a nutritionist who had enormous arms. Whenever they were together at the gym, people approached him with questions about arm exercises despite the fact that he had no real exercise background, and Jonathan, a lean endurance athlete (okay—a pencil neck) who had a Master's degree in exercise physiology, knew far more arm exercises than there are amino acids. Conversely, when people had questions pertaining to diet and losing weight, they came to Jonathan, assuming he was the man to ask, even though Mr. Biceps had a Ph.D. in nutrition. Go figure.

Joe's Uncle Harry, a short, jovial guy who worked for years as a paper salesman, had biceps like cannonballs from lifting stacks of paper all day. Whenever he visited, Joe insisted he make a muscle for Joe to squeeze. Even though he was only 5-feet, 5-inches, those prodigious melons on Harry's upper arms made him feel large. The point is that bulging biceps have long been symbols of masculine strength. Perhaps the biggest reason for this is their highly visible location. Another reason they're so identified with strength is that very often very strong men have very large arms.

As we discuss later, a lot of this has to do with who you picked as your parents (in other words, genetics). Regardless, big or not so big, there are lots of real-life reasons to have strong biceps.

Bulging Biceps

The biceps span the front of the upper arm, beginning at the upper part of the long bone of your arm (*humerus*) and ending at the point just beyond where your elbow bends. The action of the biceps is to bend the elbow and to turn your palm up toward the ceiling. This action of flexion and supination is the way you show off when you make a muscle like Joe's lovable Uncle Harry.

Why strong biceps? Because of the following reasons:

◆ Assistance with exercises for larger body parts. If your biceps are weak, they won't be of much help when performing exercises for your back.

◆ Activities of daily living. If your biceps are weak, your arms will tire while carrying your kid from the car to the bedroom, carrying packages, or using a screwdriver.

◆ They look good. Right or wrong, big biceps are seen as a sign of strength.

Here's the skinny when it comes to your biceps: these smallish muscles are involved in virtually every pulling movement you do (lat pull-downs, cable rows, and many more). As a result, you don't have to do many concentrated biceps exercises. We also recommend that you save your biceps routine for one of the last groups of exercises you do. Why? If you exhaust your biceps first, you won't get an effective work-out for your larger body parts because your biceps won't be able to withstand much more fatigue.

When doing your arm exercises, pay careful attention to your technique and posture. That means sitting and standing in an erect yet relaxed position and lifting the weight slowly through a full range of motion.

Standing Curls

This is the classic biceps exercise. If you have back problems, you should do this while standing against a wall. Even if you have a sound back, pay special attention to keeping your back straight and your elbows close to your sides.

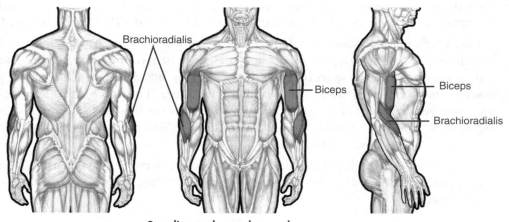

Standing curl: muscles used.

Here is how you properly perform a standing curl:

1. Grip the barbell with your palms facing outward, shoulder-width apart.
2. Stand with your feet approximately shoulder-width apart.
3. Begin with the bar resting on the front of your thighs.
4. Slowly raise the bar by bending your elbows toward your shoulders; slowly lower the bar to the front of your thighs.
5. Control the downward motion during this negative phase.

When performing a standing curl, **don't**:

◆ Rock back and forth or bend backward in an effort to get the weight up. If you must do this, you've used too much weight and should lighten the load.
◆ Let your elbows wander up as you lift.
◆ Curl the weight all the way up to your shoulders.

Do:

◆ Keep your knees slightly bent and your abdomen held tight; this will protect your back.
◆ Keep your elbows tucked in close to your body.

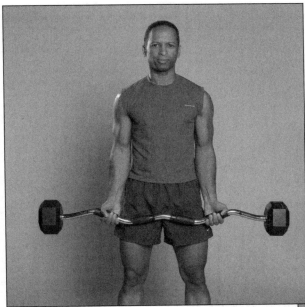

Standing curl start/finish position.

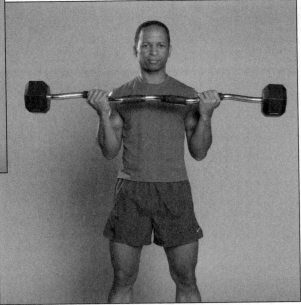

Standing curl middle position.

Dumbbell Curls

Dumbbell curls are similar to barbell curls except, well, you're using dumbbells, and instead of working both biceps at the same time, you have the option of lifting them simultaneously or alternately. Because alternating gives the muscle time to rest as the other arm is working, we prefer to work both arms together.

Here is how you properly perform a dumbbell curl:

1. Stand (or sit) with a dumbbell in each hand, your palms facing inward.
2. Slowly bend your elbow. As you do, begin to twist your wrists so your palms are facing upward.
3. Stop just short of your shoulders.
4. Slowly straighten your elbow. As you do, begin to twist your wrists so your palms are facing inward again.
5. Return to your initial starting position.

When performing a dumbbell curl, **don't:**

◆ Shrug your shoulders as you raise the dumbbells.
◆ Rock back and forth or arch your back. Again, decrease the weight if you find this happening.

Do:

◆ Keep your elbows pinned in close to your body.
◆ Keep your knees slightly bent if standing, and keep your abdomen tight, whether you are standing or sitting, to protect your back.

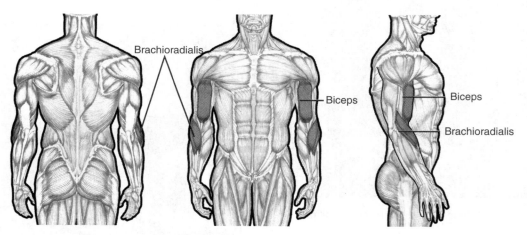

Dumbbell curl: muscles used.

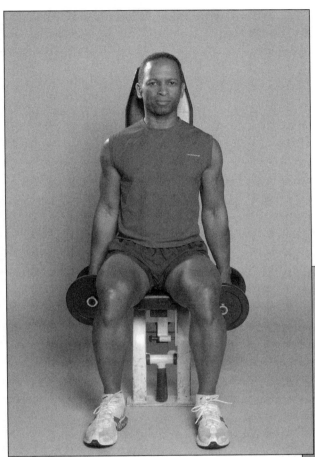

Dumbbell curl start/finish position.

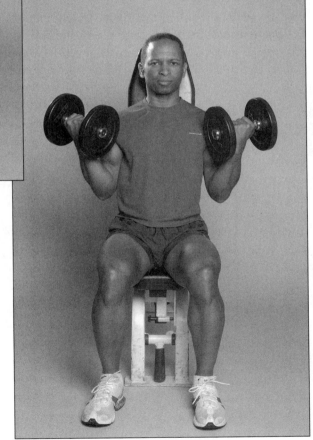

Dumbbell curl middle position.

Concentration Curls

Concentration curls are a great way to ensure that you use strict form on your curls. Because they're a little harder, you'll have to use less weight than in the previous exercise.

Here is how you properly perform a concentration curl:

1. With a dumbbell in your hand, sit on a bench, lean forward, and rest your arm on the inner part of your thigh.
2. Your palm should be facing your opposite thigh.
3. Raise the dumbbell by slowly bending to a point just short of your shoulder.
4. Lower the dumbbell by slowly straightening your elbow to the starting position.

When performing a concentration curl, **don't:**

◆ Lean or rock backward and forward in an effort to hoist the dumbbell up—you could hurt your back. If your form isn't perfect, immediately lessen the weight.

◆ Move your leg from side to side in an effort to help you lift the weight.

Do:

◆ Keep your abdomen tight and your back erect as you are leaning forward.

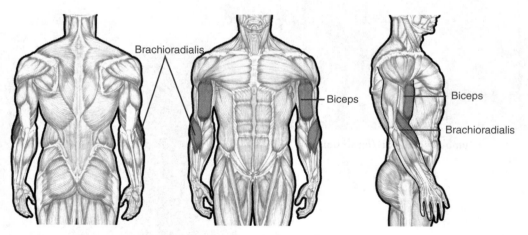

Concentration curls: muscles used.

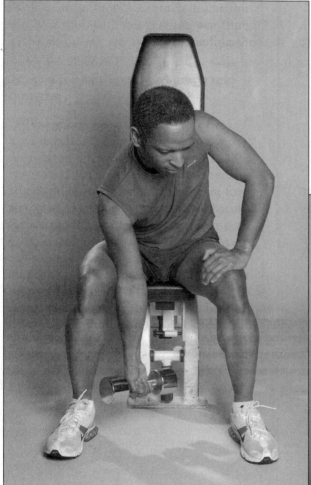

Concentration curl start/finish position.

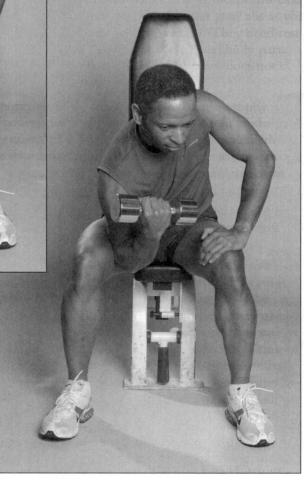

Concentration curl middle position.

Cable Curls

Cable curls are roughly equivalent to alternate dumbbell curls. They're good to do because they allow you to put constant tension on your muscle throughout the entire range of motion. Cable curls are also good because they give you a psychological change of pace.

Here is how you properly perform a cable curl:

1. Grab hold of the handle from the bottom attachment of the Cable Crossover machine. (Different, interchangeable attachments are often used on cables. For this exercise use a square-shaped handle.)

2. Be sure your palm is facing inward with your arm crossing your body slightly.

3. Stand with your feet shoulder-width apart.

4. Slowly bend your elbow, stopping just short of your shoulder.

5. Slowly straighten your elbow, stopping just short of a fully straight position. The rhythm is the same here as for every other exercise: up for a 3 count and down for a 3 count.

Spot Me

Although you will see people doing this exercise with both arms, we don't recommend it. Why? Because doing bilateral bicep cable curls will encourage you to arch your back. Unilateral bicep cable curls enable you to maintain proper posture during the exercise.

When performing a cable curl, **don't:**

◆ Lean backward to assist you with getting the weight up. If you need to do this before your last rep, reduce the weight instead.

◆ Allow the weight to bring your body forward as you lower it. If this happens, please lighten the load.

Do:

◆ Keep your abdomen tight and your knees slightly bent to protect your back.

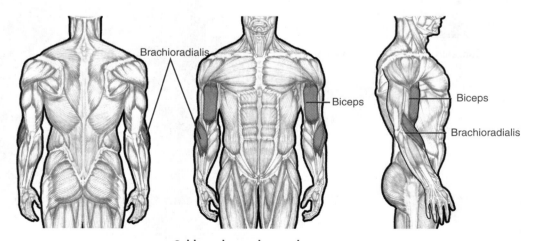

Cable curl: muscles used.

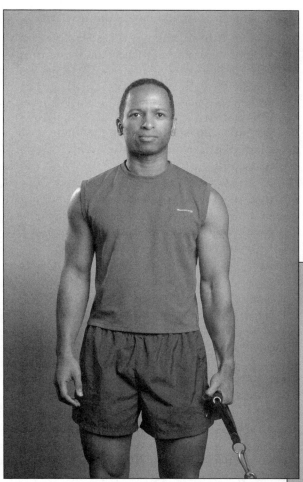

Cable curl start/finish position.

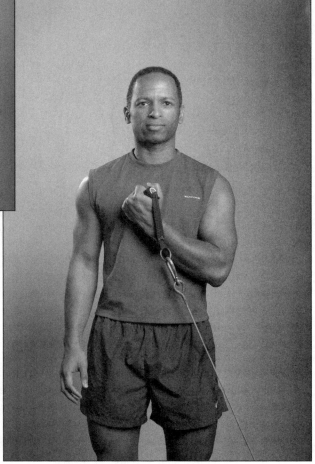

Cable curl middle position.

Machine Curls

This exercise really isolates your biceps and makes it harder for you to cheat. The setup differs between machines, but the key is to fit yourself properly to avoid cheating.

Here is how you properly perform a machine curl:

1. Sit on the seat, and place your arms on the pad. (Be sure a trainer has shown you how to adjust the machine for a proper fit. A poor fit will make the exercise less effective and place more stress on your elbow and shoulder joints.)

2. Grab hold of the handles.

3. Your feet should be flat on the floor.

4. Slowly bend your elbows as far as you can; then slowly straighten your elbows, stopping just short of a fully straight position.

When performing a machine curl, **don't:**

◆ Allow the weight to bring you up out of the seat as you lower the weight.

◆ Hold your breath.

Do:

◆ Maintain good form, 3 counts up and 3 counts down.

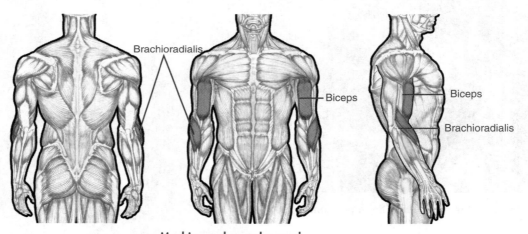

Machine curl: muscles used.

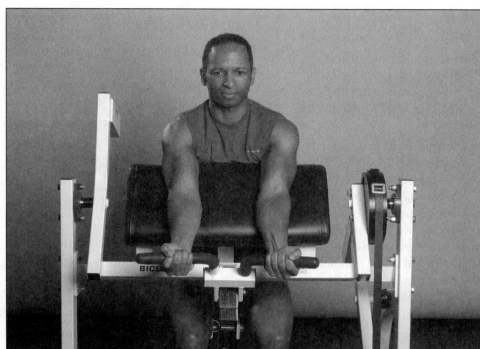

Machine curl
start/finish
position.

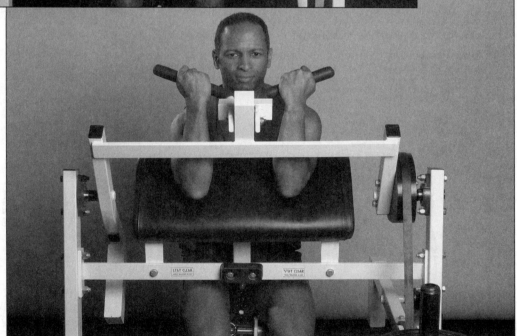

Machine curl middle position.

Triceps

You know what gives championship boxers their powerful jab? Biceps? Alas, you're wrong. It's the triceps that are responsible for that pistonlike punch that will keep your opponent (or the heavy bag) at bay.

Typically, when we train biceps, we do exercises to work the triceps as well. Located in the back of your upper arm, the triceps and biceps are neighbors who share a backyard fence. The triceps are actually made of three muscles, hence the name. Several exercises we describe in this chapter can be used to strengthen each of the three. This triangular-shaped set of muscles is involved whenever you use your shoulders or chest in pressing, pushing movements.

Why strong triceps? Because of the following reasons:

◆ They come in handy if you're forced to square off with Mike Tyson.

◆ Your prowess at pushing a shopping cart will improve.

◆ You'll have much stronger arms.

Triceps Kickbacks

The triceps kickback is a great way to isolate your triceps, but it requires strict form to be effective. You'll know you're doing it correctly when you feel the burn in the rear of your arm.

Here is how you properly perform a triceps kickback:

1. Place one knee and one hand on the bench for support.
2. Slightly bend your standing leg.
3. Your working arm should be bent 90° at your shoulder and 90° at your elbow.
4. Keep your arm close to your side. To gain the full benefit from this exercise, it's important to keep your upper arm parallel to the ground. Pay strict attention to your form.
5. Slowly straighten your elbow, and return to the starting position.

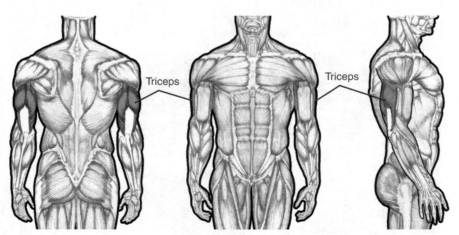

Triceps kickback: muscles used.

When performing a triceps kickback, **don't**:

◆ Allow your back to sag.

◆ Shift your body back and forth in an effort to get the weight up.

◆ Let your upper arm drop—keep it parallel to the ground throughout the range of motion.

Do:

◆ Keep your back straight and your abdomen tight.

◆ Keep your eyes fixed on the bench. Looking up or sideways can put stress on your neck.

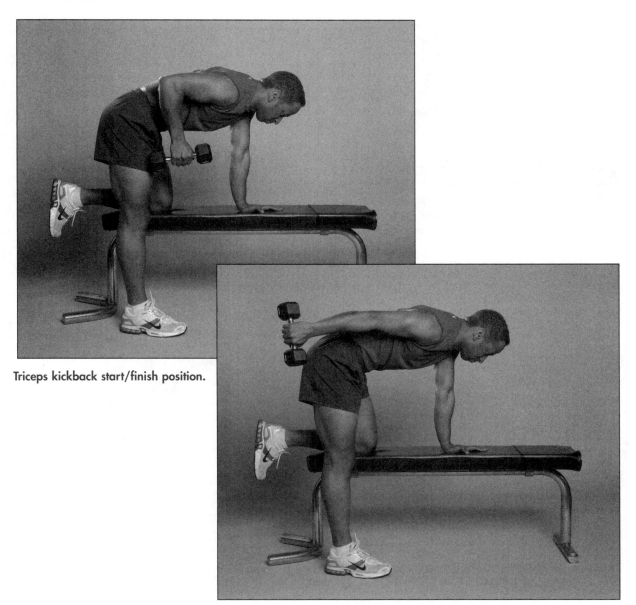

Triceps kickback start/finish position.

Triceps kickback middle position.

French Curls

We're not sure why this particular exercise is identified with France, but feel free to do it regardless of your nationality. It's an excellent way to work your triceps.

Here is how you properly perform a French curl:

1. While standing or sitting, raise the dumbbell overhead and bend your elbow to a point where you are feeling a stretch in your triceps.
2. Begin to straighten your elbow, and slowly return to your initial starting position.

Weight a Minute

Be careful if you have been diagnosed with shoulder impingement syndrome (an abnormal squeezing of the structures within the shoulder joint). French curls can worsen the condition.

When performing a French curl, **don't:**

◆ Shift your body from side to side in an effort to raise the weight.
◆ Snap or lock your elbow upon straightening it.
◆ Allow the weight to fall rapidly to the starting position.

Do:

◆ Keep your abdomen tight, whether sitting or standing.
◆ Concentrate on your triceps and move gently through a full range of motion.

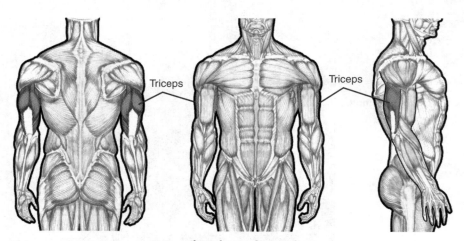

Triceps   Triceps

French curl: muscles used.

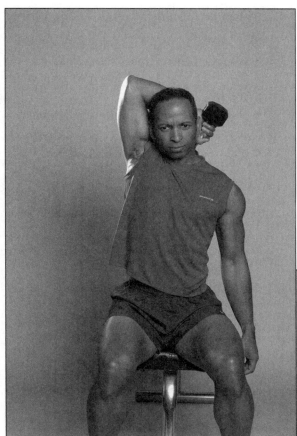

French curl start/finish position.

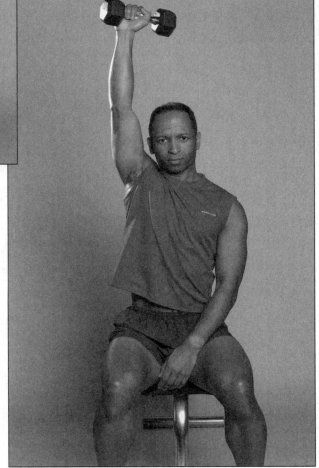

French curl middle position.

Pushdowns

It's important to push hard at the bottom of the repetition to tighten (contract) your triceps. You can use either a rope or bar attachment to perform this exercise; the rope is the harder of the two, and you will typically use less weight than with the bar.

Here is how you properly perform a pushdown:

1. Grab hold of the pushdown bar. Your elbows should be bent to 90° and held close to your side.

2. Slowly straighten your elbows, and return to your initial starting position.

When performing a pushdown, **don't**:

◆ Lean forward as you push down the weight. This reduces the isolation from the triceps and transfers it to your whole body.

◆ Lock your elbows in the straightened position.

◆ Allow the weight to fall rapidly.

Do:

◆ Keep your abdomen tight and your back erect.

◆ Keep your head facing forward, not down or sideways.

◆ Keep your elbows close to your side.

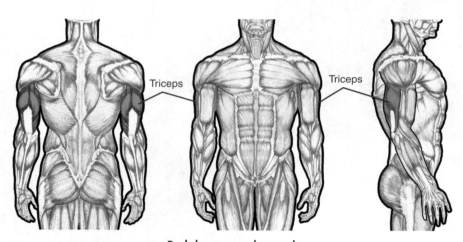

Pushdown: muscles used.

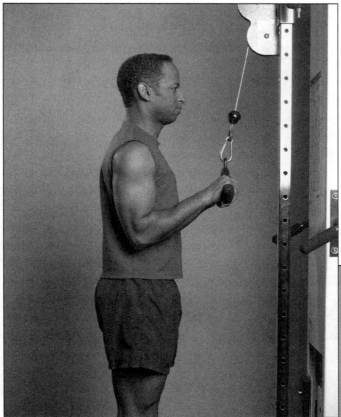

Pushdown start/finish position.

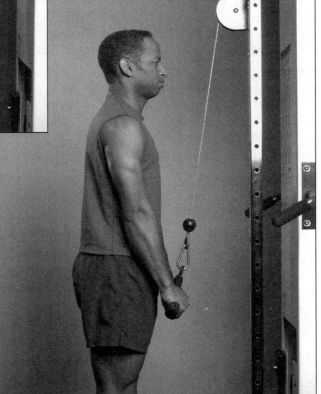

Pushdown middle position.

Wrist Not, Want Not

The muscles that work to bend and straighten your wrists actually originate at the elbow. In case you were curious, the muscles that bend (flex) the wrist originate on the inner part of the elbow. The muscles that straighten (extend) the wrist originate on the outer aspect of the elbow.

Why strong wrists? Because of the following reasons:

◆ Weak wrist muscles can lead to golfer's elbow (*medial epicondylitis*) or tennis elbow (*lateral epicondylitis*). These injuries affect the pros as well as weekend warriors like you and me.

◆ Everyday activities like carrying heavy grocery bags or luggage can put strain on these muscles. In fact, people who use a screwdriver frequently suffer from tendinitis.

◆ If you care to embark on a career as a professional arm wrestler, you'll need strong wrists.

The best medicine is the preventive kind, which is why strengthening your wrists is important. A good way to avoid injuring your wrists is to do the following exercises.

Weight a Minute

If you have carpal tunnel syndrome, do not perform these exercises, because they're likely to aggravate it. This condition is often caused by repetitive activities done with improper body mechanics, such as typing with your wrists in an extended position (they should be neutral) or repetitive squeezing activities (such as what a cake decorator would do when decorating a cake). The median nerve swells and is unable to pass comfortably through the small bones in your wrist (carpals). Symptoms of carpal tunnel syndrome are numbness, tingling, or a sharp, shooting pain into your hand.

Wrist Flexion

Here is how you properly perform wrist flexion:

1. Lean forward.
2. Place your forearms on your thighs. The dumbbell should be held in a position past your knees with your palm up.
3. Allow your wrist to bend as far back as you comfortably can.
4. Slowly bend your wrist up as far as you can; then return to the initial starting position.

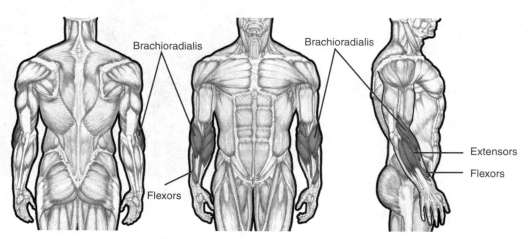

Wrist flexion/extension: muscles used.

Wrist Extension

Perform this exercise the same as you would the wrist flexion, except your palms should be facing down (instead of up).

When performing wrist flexion and extension, **don't:**

◆ Perform the movements rapidly in either direction.

Do:

◆ Keep your abdomen tight and your back erect.

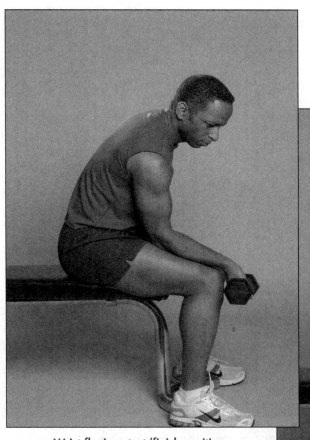

Wrist flexion start/finish position.

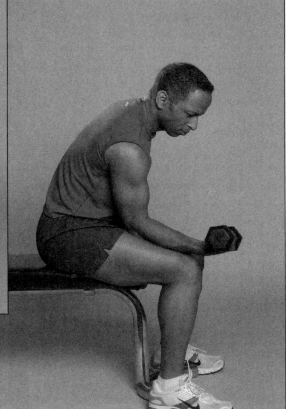

Wrist flexion middle position.

In This Chapter

- ◆ Comparing abs versus flab
- ◆ Understanding the rectus abdominis
- ◆ Losing the midsection myths
- ◆ Joining the washboard world

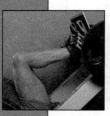 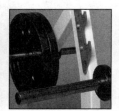 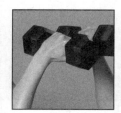 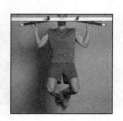 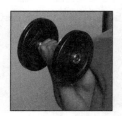 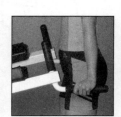

Chapter 12

Gut Buster

Here's a bit of abdominal irony to ponder: as a nation, we seem to loathe fat people even though we're the most overweight nation in the Western world. A portly belly might have been a sign of prosperity in the Far East, but in our culture, a flat stomach is a prized possession, despite the fact that most people refuse to do what it takes to get there.

Socioeconomic implications aside, there are several solid reasons to build a washboard stomach:

◆ It looks good.
◆ It will make you feel better, especially if you have an ailing back.
◆ You'll be stronger in the weight room and on the playing field.
◆ You may become a famous underwear model.

Before we give you the lowdown on building up your midsection, let's review our anatomy. The first, and most common, mistake is referring to the abdominals (the "abs") as "the stomach." The abs are the muscles in your midsection; your stomach is the organ that processes the food you consume. Ab exercises have traditionally included sit-ups and leg lifts; stomach exercises include dining in a French restaurant.

Your abdominals consist of four muscles:

◆ The *rectus abdominis*, the largest muscle in the abs, is a wide, flat sheet of muscle that runs from just under the lower part of your chest to just below your belly button. When you do abdominal crunches, the old rectus abdominis muscle is hard at work. (For more on crunches, read on.) It also keeps your spine from slip-sliding around when you're exercising other body parts.

◆ The *internal obliques* and *external obliques*, which run diagonally along your sides, not only assist the rectus in curling the spine, but also twist and bend your upper body. These muscles are central in any sport involving upper body rotation—golf, baseball, kayaking, and many more—and they are integral in a strengthening program, especially if you have a bad back. Why? These muscles wrap around your waist and, when properly conditioned, provide much-needed support for your lower back. In essence, the obliques are the world's most comfortable, form-fitting girdle.

◆ The *transversus abdominis*, which sounds like a phrase from a Latin Mass, is the deepest of all the muscles in your abs. Located directly below the rectus abdominis, it is called into action when you sneeze, cough, or exhale forcefully. There are no specific exercises you can do to target this muscle, but you can strengthen the transversus abdominis by forcefully exhaling during the positive phase of your ab exercises.

Feel the Burn

As we've mentioned, having strong abs significantly helps you get rid of lower back pain. Try this: sit in a chair. Hold your abs tight. Now let them go. Did you note a difference in your posture? You see, your abs are what keep your pelvis in a neutral position. When your abs are weak, your pelvis has a tendency to tilt forward, increasing the inward curve of your lumbar spine. This, of course, will throw the rest of your spine out of whack as well. All you have to do to see what we're talking about is check out the exaggerated curve of someone with a sizeable beer belly. Contrast that, say, with the posture of an athlete such as an Olympic gymnast, and you can begin to see the relationship between strong abs, good posture, and improved athletic performance.

Perhaps because there's so much discussion and even obsession with our bulging waistlines, there's a lot of misinformation surrounding the abs that we'd like to clear up.

Here are a few of the most common mid-section myths:

◆ **"If I work my abs, I'll get rid of my love handles."** This is the one we hear most often. However, you can do 5,000 sit-ups a day, and if you still have excess adipose tissue (a fancy medical term for *fat*), you'll have really strong abs obscured by your love handles. Because the muscle lies beneath the fat, if you consume more calories than you burn, these powerful muscles will function efficiently but not be revealed to the public at large. In other words, strong abs and love handles have nothing to do with each other. Want to lose the excess baggage? Eat less and do more cardiovascular exercise.

◆ **"I need to do 500 crunches a day to get my abs in really great shape."** In fact, if you can do 500 crunches a day, you're either a Navy SEAL in training or doing something quite wrong. Done correctly, 10 to 25 repetitions for 3 sets is more than enough to get the job done. Why waste your time by doing so many, especially if you do them incorrectly?

◆ **"I do my abs every day for maximum benefit."** This is another line we hear a lot in the gym. The abs can be worked more than your chest or biceps, for example, but you should treat your abs as you treat any other muscles. They need rest just like any other stressed body part. Working them more often does not improve results.

Crunches

If you're stuck on a desert island with just one ab exercise, crunches are the one. Done properly, you're bound to feel a nice burn in no time flat.

Here is how you properly perform a crunch:

1. Lie on a mat with your knees bent and your feet on the floor. Depending on your level of fitness, you can place your arms in any of the three following positions:

   Beginner: With your arms straight at your sides and your fingers pointing toward your knees.

   Intermediate: With your arms crossed over your chest.

   Advanced: With your elbows bent and your fingers overlapping behind your neck.

2. Tighten your stomach muscles, and slowly curl your torso up until your shoulder blades are off the floor.

3. Slowly return to your starting position without completely relaxing on the floor.

Initially the exercise may feel rather easy; however, after several reps, you should begin to feel a burn in the upper third of your abs.

When performing a crunch, **don't:**

◆ Bend your neck as you curl into the crunch position. This is the biggest reason that people who do a lot of ab work complain. Imagine having a softball between your chin and your chest.

◆ Draw your elbows in. You're trying to lift your torso, not flap your elbows.

◆ Bring your torso up past 30°.

Do:

◆ Keep your head and neck in a neutral position; the less stress on your neck, the better.

◆ Be sure you curl as you lift.

◆ Focus your attention on the top section of your abdominals. Let them—and not any other part of your upper body—do the work.

◆ Keep your lower back pressed against the floor at all times.

Weight a Minute

Be sure not to "throw" your head forward when doing crunches. To avoid causing neck pain, your hands should support your head and you should maintain space between your chin and your chest.

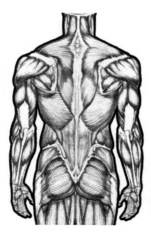
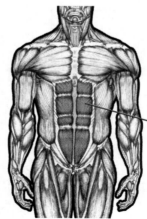
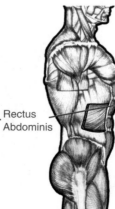

Rectus Abdominis

Crunches: muscles used.

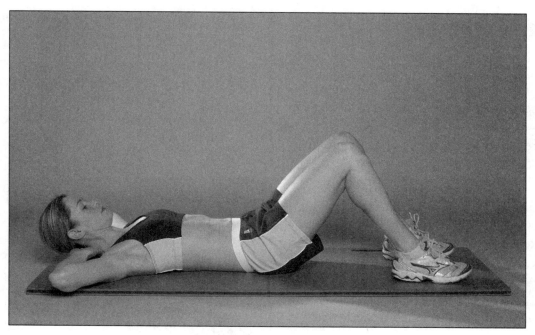

Crunch start/finish position.

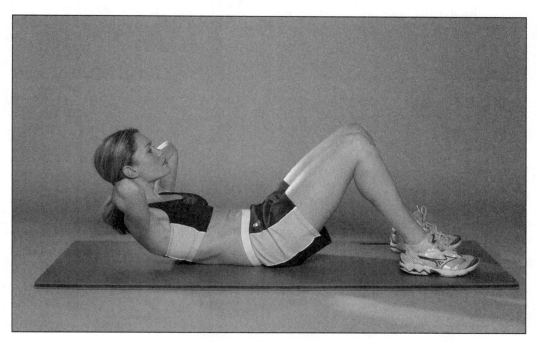

Crunch middle position.

Reverse Crunches

Here's a tricky one that takes some time to get used to. It's not nearly as impressive-looking as some of the crazy leg lifts and other things you'll see people doing in an effort to strengthen their lower abs, but it's far more safe and effective.

Here is how you properly perform a reverse crunch:

1. Lie on a mat with your legs up and your knees slightly bent. In the starting position, you'll look like a big letter L.
2. Rest your arms on the floor at your sides.
3. Keep your head on the mat, and tighten your abdominals.
4. Lift your butt off the floor so your legs go up and slightly backward toward your head.
5. Hold this position for a second, and slowly return to the starting position.

When performing a reverse crunch, **don't**:

◆ Roll your hips so your back comes off the mat.
◆ Tighten your shoulders or involve any upper body movement.
◆ Hold your breath. (People always seem to on this exercise.)

Do:

◆ Keep the movement small—no need to roll back, too.
◆ Keep the movement smooth.
◆ Isolate the muscle by concentrating on the lower section of your abs.

Spot Me

Because your abdominal muscles assist when you forcefully exhale, breathing out during the positive phase of your ab exercises helps you get an even better contraction.

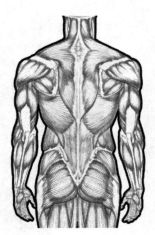
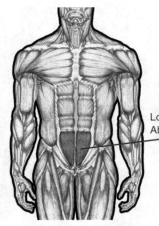
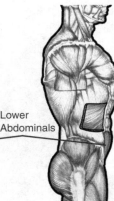

Lower
Abdominals

Reverse crunches: muscles used.

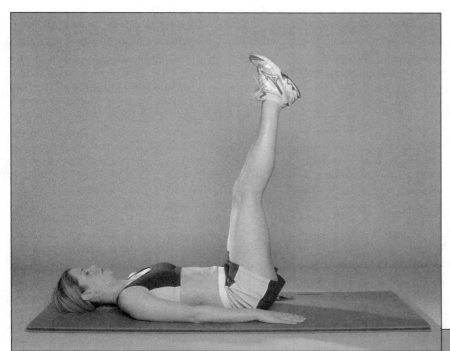

**Reverse crunch
start/finish position.**

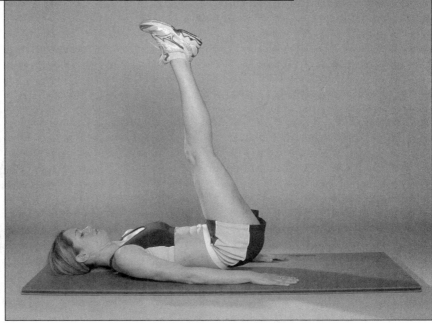

Reverse crunch middle position.

Ball Crunches

The ball crunch is a variation on the standard crunch and is performed on an oversized orb called a *Swiss Ball* or *Stability Ball*. The ball is obviously less stable than a mat and forces you to use small stabilizing muscles in your midsection to help maintain balance.

Here's the drill:

1. Sit on the high section of the ball with your feet flat on the floor and hip width apart. Lay back on the ball. Place your hands in the same position as in the crunch.

2. Contract your abdominal muscles, and raise your torso off the ball until your shoulder blades and mid-back are clear.

3. Slowly lower yourself back onto the ball, keeping your abs tight at all times.

The form is largely the same as with the crunch, although the range of motion is great.

When doing the ball crunch, **don't:**

◆ Bounce off the ball at the bottom.
◆ Thrust your head forward.

Do:

◆ Contract your abs when lifting and lowering.
◆ Keep your feet on the floor.

Bar Talk

Swiss Balls or **Stability Balls** are large, inflatable rubber balls used for abdominal and other exercises. The come in different sizes, with a 55-inch diameter recommended for those under 5 feet, 5 inches; 65 inches for those up to 6 feet tall; and 75 inches for people taller than 6 feet.

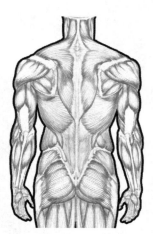
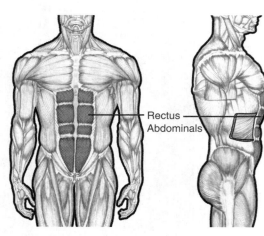

Rectus Abdominals

Ball crunches: muscles used.

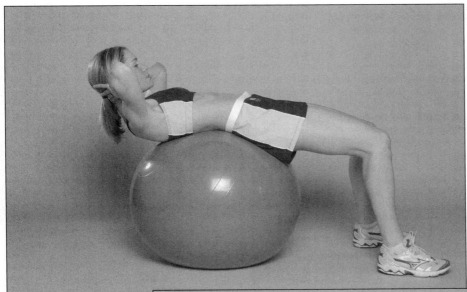

Ball crunch start/finish position.

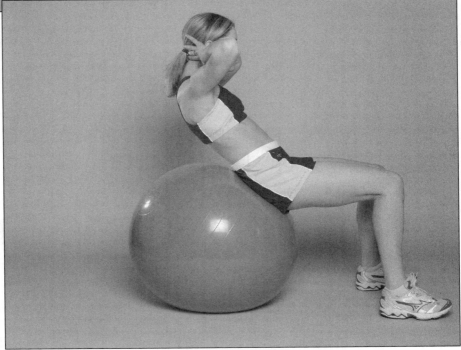

Ball crunch middle position.

Oblique Crunches

Here's another one that's commonly abused in the gym. Focus on moving your shoulder toward your opposite knee. Avoid the temptation to move your elbow in or your knee back.

Here's how you properly perform an oblique crunch:

1. Lie on a mat with your left leg bent and your foot flat on the floor.
2. Place your right ankle so it rests on top of your left knee.
3. Position your left hand behind your neck, and keep your right arm outstretched.
4. Slowly curl up and twist toward your right knee.

5. Hold that position for a second and then slowly return to the starting position.
6. Switch legs and arms, and repeat on the other side.

When performing an oblique crunch, **don't**:

◆ Bend your head with your hand.
◆ Merely move your elbow to your knee.

Do:

◆ Curl and twist your shoulder toward your opposite knee.
◆ Keep the movement slow and controlled.

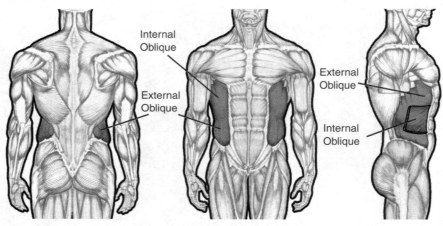

Oblique crunches: muscles used.

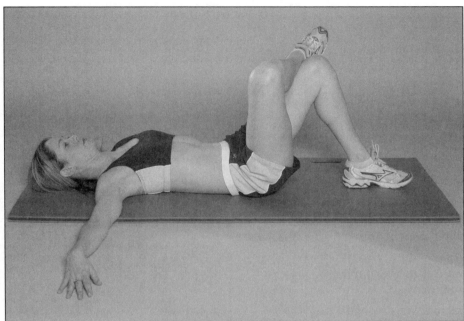

Oblique crunch
start/finish position.

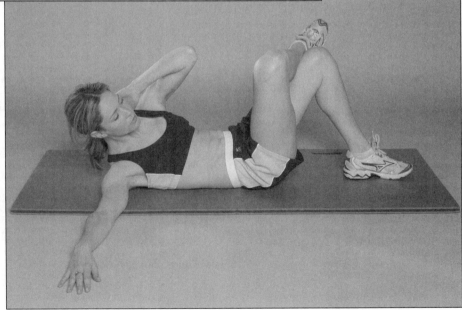

Oblique crunch middle position.

Side Obliques

Here's an alternative to the previous exercise. Use it to break up the monotony whenever you please. If you choose this exercise, be sure to keep your knees over to the side to keep the focus on your obliques.

Here is how you properly perform a side oblique:

1. Lie on a mat on your right side with your knees bent.
2. Place both hands behind your neck, and keep your head looking straight at the ceiling.
3. Use your oblique muscles to lift your upper body slightly off the mat.
4. Hold yourself off the mat for a second and then return to your starting position.

When performing a side oblique, **don't:**

◆ Bend your neck to the side as you lift your torso off the mat.

Do:

◆ Keep your shoulder and head going straight toward the ceiling.
◆ Be sure your knees stay over to the side.

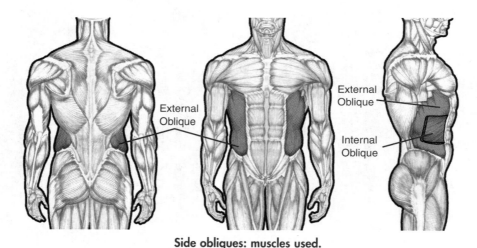

Side obliques: muscles used.

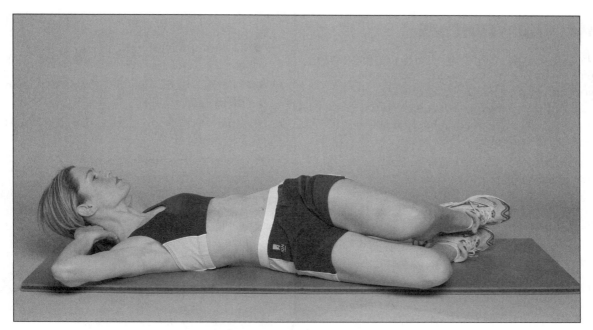

Side oblique start/finish position.

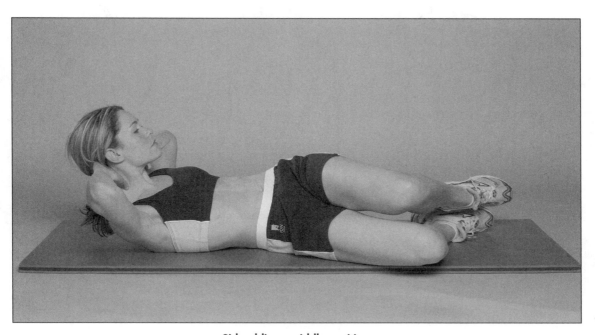

Side oblique middle position.

Machine Crunches

To isolate your abdomen, slowly move the arm pad toward your knees using the muscles in your upper abs. Pause for a second at the bottom of the repetition, and return to the starting position without completely releasing the tension in your abs.

Here is how you properly perform a machine crunch:

1. Sit on the seat, and fasten the belt if one is provided.
2. Place your arms on top of the arm pad.
3. Slowly tighten your abdominal muscles, curling your torso forward. As you do this, you'll be bringing the arm pad toward your thighs.

When performing a machine crunch, **don't:**

◆ Use too much weight so your hips are lifted off the seat.
◆ Let the weights you're lifting slam down on the stack.
◆ Arch your back as you return to the starting position.
◆ Focus on pushing the arm pad down; rather, concentrate on curling your abdomen.

Do:

◆ Keep constant tension on your abdominals as you perform the exercise.

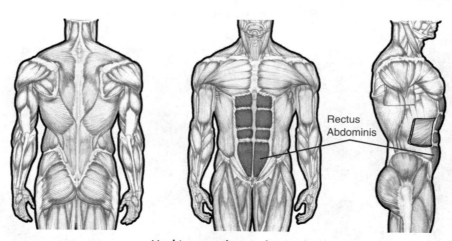

Rectus Abdominis

Machine crunch: muscles used.

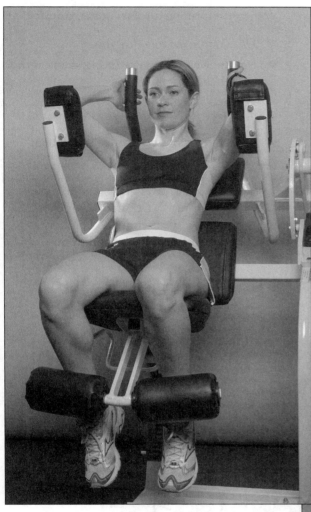

Machine crunch start/finish position.

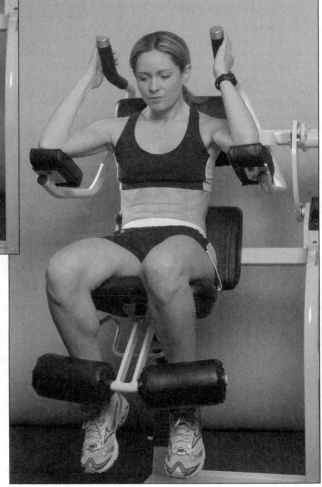

Machine crunch middle position.

Rotary Torso

This machine does a great job of isolating the obliques. Still, we're not big fans of this machine unless you're careful to use strict form. Do it smoothly and you'll be fine; how-ever, constant, weighted, and uncontrolled rotation can cause your back more harm than the good it will do for your abs.

Here is how you properly perform a rotary torso:

1. Sit on the seat.
2. Position your arms behind each arm pad. Get ready to twist like a young Elvis.
3. Slowly twist your body until you can twist no farther.
4. Pause for a second, and slowly return to the starting position.
5. Repeat on the other side.

When performing a rotary torso, **don't:**

◆ Use your arms to assist you.
◆ Let the weights you're lifting slam on the stack below.

Do:

◆ Maintain a slow, controlled movement throughout the rotation.

People with back problems shouldn't use this machine. Instead, stick with floor exercises where you have greater control. The twisting motion can aggravate a back condition.

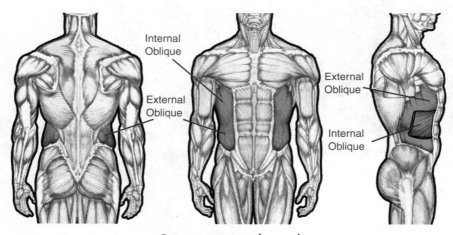

Rotary torso: muscles used.

Internal Oblique

External Oblique

External Oblique

Internal Oblique

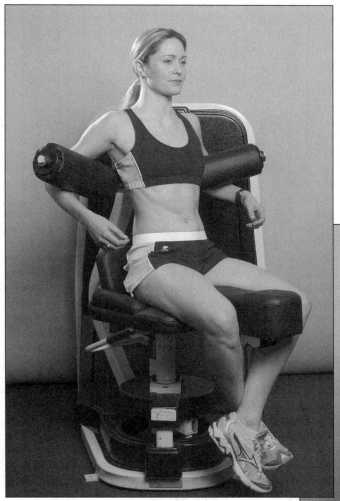

Rotary torso start/finish position.

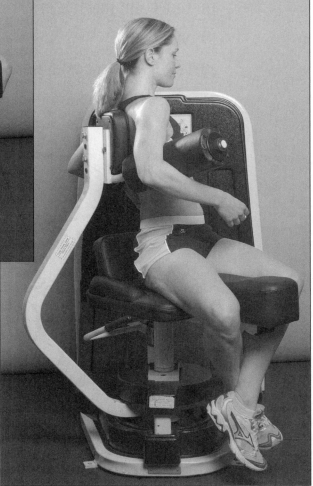

Rotary torso middle position.

In This Part

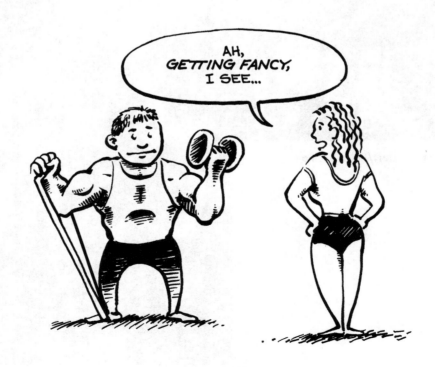

Leaner and Meaner

Now that you've learned the nuances of the equipment, the exercises, and the philosophy behind working out, in Part 3, we show you how to put it all together. We give you guidelines on which exercises to include in your routine depending on your goals and time constraints, and what to do if things aren't working out the way you expected.

In This Chapter

◆ Putting it all together

◆ Knowing when sore is good

◆ Understanding when too much is bad

◆ Being bored no more

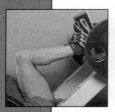 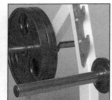 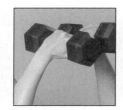 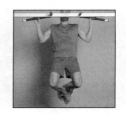 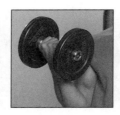 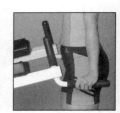

Chapter **13**

Get With the Program

You've read this far, and you no doubt know more than you ever wanted to know about form, safety, sets, and reps, as well as a slew of fancy words that ensure you know the difference between your lats and your pecs. In addition, you're now familiar with the mechanics of a host of exercises to keep you busy until the next millennium. What you might not know, however, is how to put it all together. Having all the ingredients for a soufflé is one thing; knowing how to assemble them is another. In this and in the ensuing chapters, we show you how to take the information we've discussed thus far and use it to build a workout routine fit for a hungry king.

As we've mentioned, talk to a dozen fitness experts, and you're liable to get half a dozen or more opinions on how much to lift, how often, and more. Although virtually everyone will tell you to progress from larger muscles to smaller muscles, the wide variety of opinions can be quite confusing. We can't say everyone who dares to disagree with us has a head full of iron, but we can tell you that if you follow what we suggest in this and the chapters that follow, you'll get stronger, as well as look and feel better. If you're skeptical, try one of the following routines and see for yourself.

Finally, we realize all gyms are not created equal. As a result, you may not have all the equipment we demonstrated at your disposal. To account for this athletic inequity, we've included a few different basic workout plans to get you started.

What to Do

When you look over the programs in this chapter, your first reaction may be that there are not a whole lot of exercises included. There's a reason for this. Because we're asking you to work hard and exhibit perfect form on each, as a trade-off, we won't ask you to do a lot of exercises. After all, it's only human that your concentration and willpower will falter if you have to do an endless series of exercises each time out. As we promised throughout the book, working out won't take you all day, and we meant it.

These basic routines shouldn't take more than 45 minutes each. That includes about 1 minute for each of the exercises and 2 minutes off between each set. That's not a significant investment in time, but if you do these routines faithfully—with effort and concentration—you'll get stronger. As you can see from the following chart, we've imitated a Chinese menu (one from the first column; one from the second column) and tried to give you the option of deciding between freeweights or machine exercises whenever possible. Depending on your preference and the availability of any one machine or freeweight apparatus, there's no need to stick with one or the other exclusively.

Whenever you see an exercise highlighted in **bold,** that means we want you to do a light warm-up set with about half your normal weight before moving on to your regular set of these exercises. Remember to aim for sets of 10 to 12 reps with a 3-second positive and 3-second negative, with a 1-second pause between. In other words, lifting the weight will take 3 seconds, the downward phase will take 3 seconds, and so on until the set is done. Take 2 minutes between exercises. You can take less time if you care to, but try hard not to take more. If you do, that 45-minute figure will creep over the 1-hour mark.

Here's a chart to help you pick one of the following exercises from the machine column and/or freeweight column. Feel free to mix it up—use some freeweight exercises and some machines if you like. Work your way from the top of the list down to the bottom.

Mix-and-Match Machines and Freeweights

Muscle	Machine Exercise	Freeweight Exercise
Glutes, quads, hamstrings	**Leg press**	**Lunges**
Quads	Leg extension	
Hamstrings	Leg curl	
Gastroc (calves)	Standing toe raise	
Lats	**Lat pull-down**	**Pull-ups** (assisted, if necessary)
Traps	Shrug	
Pecs	**Chest press**	**Bench press**
Flye	Pec deck	
Delts	Shoulder press	Dumbbell military press
	Lateral raise	Lateral raise
Biceps	Biceps machine	Seated dumbbell curl
Triceps	Triceps pushdown	French curl
Abs	Abdominal machine	Crunches
Obliques	Rotary torso	Oblique crunches
Lower back	Back raise	

Keeping Track

Your main goal during the first few weeks is to learn to do the exercises properly. At the same time, it's important that you keep track of what you're doing. That's where a workout log comes in. We don't want to make this seem like preparing your income taxes. However, not only will keeping accurate records of your workouts help you track your progress, it's also a great way to figure out what to do when you hit a plateau. Getting stronger requires that you overload your muscles; as a result it's key that you know what you've done in previous workouts. If you're anything like us, you'll actually find it fun to see how much progress you've made in a relatively short amount of time.

Your workout log should list everything you've done that day in the gym—your choice of exercises, how much weight, how many reps—as well as the height of the seat on the machines you're using. It's also a good idea to note how you were feeling on that day, your body weight, and any other relevant facts. In time, you'll see that this physical record is a diary that will accurately reflect the relationship between your mental, physical, and emotional lives. In fact, the more carefully you note the impact of outside factors on your lifting, the more you're likely to see a powerful relationship between how all facets of your life affect your weight training.

I'm Late! I'm Late!

Of course, in this busy world where time is often money, even 45 minutes can seem like too much time to spare. If that's the case for you, don't worry. It's far better to work out just a little than not at all. Let's say you want to squeeze in a workout at lunch and still have time to shower and grab a bite. Or perhaps you want to run a couple miles and have just 20 minutes or so to lift afterward. No matter; we'll give you a condensed workout to keep you on track.

These shorter workouts are not as thorough as the longer versions, and they're better suited to maintaining strength rather than getting you stronger, but they take care of the basics. Just as important, they ensure you won't lose fitness.

The shorter workout is essentially the same as the longer one. The biggest difference is that each of these exercises is a *multijoint* or *compound movement*, meaning you'll be working at least two joints, which means you'll be working more muscles during any one lift. *Single-joint* or *isolation movements* like the flye (chest) or lateral raise (shoulder) are great, but you don't cover as much ground with each exercise.

Bar Talk

Multijoint or **compound movements** are exercises that involve two or more joints. **Single-joint** or **isolation movements** use only one. Compound movements like the bench press or squat use more musculature and generally result in the weight moving in a fairly straight line, whereas isolation moves like the flye or leg extension focus on a specific muscle and usually have a rotary movement.

Perform a light warm-up set of the bold exercises. Reduce your recovery time between sets from 2 minutes to 1. Done correctly, you're in and out in less than 15 minutes. Remember that just because you're in a hurry, it doesn't mean your reps should be performed quickly. Focus on proper form, and get as much out of each and every rep as you can. The key here is intensity.

The following table can be your quickie guide to a great 15-minute workout.

15-Minute Workout

Muscle	Exercise
Glutes, hamstrings, quads	**Leg press**
Lats	**Lat pull-down or pull-ups**
Pecs	**Bench press or dips**
Traps	Upright rows
Delts	Shoulder press
Abs	Crunches

Progress Report

Let's say you've done every rep of every set with perfect form. Let's also assume you warm up and stretch religiously, and your nutrition is as pure as a field of soybeans. What you will discover, no doubt, is that no matter how slowly you started your program, you've had your share of aches and pains. If you're wondering if this is normal, the answer is "yes." The bottom line is that although we'll do everything we can to help you avoid injuries, muscle soreness is a natural consequence of a new weight-lifting program.

Whenever you introduce a new activity to your body, you experience what we will call growing pains. This is a natural consequence as your muscles, tendons, and ligaments adapt to the new stresses and strains of muscular overload. In fact, even someone who is ridiculously fit will be sore if they do a new routine with any intensity. What we want you to be able to do is differentiate between *good* hurt and *bad* hurt. Good hurt you can work through; bad hurt is a sure signal to stop immediately.

There are two types of soreness you're likely to experience during weight training: acute soreness—the discomfort you feel during and right after a set—and a more gradual, duller ache that comes on in the days after you lift.

The Burn

In gym parlance, acute soreness is referred to as the "burn." Typically, it occurs during and immediately following exercise. When you're completing the last few reps of a set, your muscles are working hard. As the muscle is taxed, it actually presses against your arteries and cuts off blood flow. (This is the rough equivalent of having an inflated cuff on when you're having your blood pressure taken.) As a result, lactic acid, a byproduct of anaerobic activity, accumulates. This combination of lactic acid and blood flow occlusion is what is thought to cause momentary muscle failure. Got that? The miracle of the human body is that within a few seconds of the end of the set, the burn dissipates as the muscle is engorged with even more blood than usual to compensate for what was lost during the set. This process is what causes the temporary (but ego-boosting) "pump" phenomenon.

The DOMS

Delayed onset muscle soreness (DOMS) refers to pain and soreness that occurs 24 to 48 hours after exercise. DOMS is due to the microscopic muscle damage that takes place when you lift. The eccentric or negative phase of the exercise contributes more than its fair share to this soreness—especially if you use extra weight for the negatives (a technique we'll describe in Chapter 15). Usually, you'll feel the beginning of DOMS the day after you lift; however, it often reaches its peak at about 48 hours after the fact. Putting ice on the affected area can help reduce some of the edema (or retention of water) at the site and help alleviate the pain. The soreness should start to ease after that and last no more than 3 to 4 days. If the pain lasts significantly longer or becomes worse, we suggest you see a physician.

Spot Me

Though we've given you a number of reasons why you should stretch, alleviating delayed onset muscle soreness is not one of them. Despite gym lore, stretching doesn't speed your recovery from DOMS. Studies have shown that while increased flexibility may help prevent or decrease the incidence of soreness in the first place, after you're sore, stretching isn't going to help.

That Hurts!

A burn during a set and soreness afterward is as common as a pigeon in a park. Although the term *good pain* may be a classic oxymoron, there certainly are normal pains associated with the weight-lifting game. Of course, some types of pain are not normal and shouldn't be taken lightly. In fact, unless you've been doing it a long while, the old bromide of "No pain, no gain" is generally considered passé and counterproductive.

Here's the bottom line: any sharp and shooting pain is bad, no matter where it occurs. Such an acute sensation is indicative of nerve pain and should send a warning that's attended to immediately. Pain that occurs in any of your joints (shoulder, elbow, wrist, hip, knee, or ankle) is also a red flag. As we've stressed all along, be mindful of your form and of the amount of weight you're lifting.

Flex Facts

Lactic acid is usually to blame when you feel a burning sensation during your lift or while sprinting to catch a bus, but it's just an innocent bystander when it comes to DOMS. Even after a brutal workout, your lactic acid levels are back to normal within a couple hours of a workout.

If your form is not sound, you are putting additional stress on your joints simply because you are putting your body in a position it doesn't want to be in. This means that even if you were performing the exercise with just your body weight, you would experience some pain and discomfort. Add a barbell to the equation, and you're bound to aggravate the situation. It sounds so simple, but time and time again we see people lifting heavy weights with chronically injured joints. Determination clearly has a place in the gym, but when it's misapplied, it's a sure way to court serious injury.

Weight a Minute

A burning sensation is normal during a challenging set of weight lifting, and soreness over the next couple days is not unusual. However, any sharp or shooting pain while lifting is a red flag to stop immediately. If this occurs, never try to fight through such pain. Review your form to be sure you're not doing anything wrong. If your form isn't at fault, try another exercise that works the same body part.

Let's take a look at a couple broad categories and discuss how to best treat them.

Pulls and Strains

Minor muscle pulls or muscle *strains* are a common injury associated with weight lifting. With careful attention to proper technique and caution against using too much weight, strains can usually be avoided.

Sprains are another common injury, though they are usually avoidable. Moderate strains and sprains are usually treated in the same way, with rest, ice, compression, and elevation, or RICE. Here are the specifics:

- **Rest.** Eliminates the demands on the affected area. If you can't rest it entirely, at least modify it as much as possible. (That would be MICE.)
- **Ice.** Decreases swelling, pain, and circulation.
- **Compression.** Limits swelling with the pressure of a bandage.
- **Elevation.** Reduces or limits swelling by reducing blood flow to injured area.

Bar Talk

A muscle **strain** or pull is a trauma to the muscle or tendon caused by excessive contraction or stretching. **Sprains** are damage to ligaments (ligaments are the connective tissue between bones) accompanied by swelling and sometimes by discoloration.

Overtraining

Overtraining can be another source of aches and pains. It's also a factor that may inhibit muscular strength gains. Symptoms of overtraining include the following:

- Chronic fatigue
- Appetite disorders
- Sleeplessness
- Depression
- Anger
- Substantial weight gain or loss
- Protracted muscle soreness
- Elevated resting heart rate
- Lack of progress in muscular strength

If you are experiencing any of these symptoms with your weight-lifting program, perhaps you began too ambitiously. In our experience, the two most common symptoms of overtraining are an uncomfortable night's sleep and moodiness.

Listen to your body, rest, and begin again at a more modest pace.

Bar Talk

Overtraining occurs when you train without allowing sufficient recovery between workouts or do too much too fast. Sometimes it rears its ugly head with physical symptoms, and sometimes it's mental. Usually a couple extra days off will help remedy the situation.

If you've been lifting consistently, don't worry that a few extra days off will hurt your strength. Many of Jonathan's most dedicated clients travel quite a bit—either for work or for pleasure. Oftentimes, he'll tell them to relax and not work out on the road. Much to their surprise, they actually benefit from the short break, and they're stronger than ever when they return.

When she was competing as a powerlifter, our sage expert Deidre was a poster child for overtraining. Not only did she not stretch, Deidre also worked out *every single day*, whether it was lifting weights or doing aerobics. She looked great, but she was an achy mess most of the time, especially in the morning when she struggled to get out of bed with a chronically sore lower back. During her last year of competition in 1997, she was hurt more often than not and was frequently depressed and disagreeable. If her coach said the sky was up, she'd argue otherwise. Such is the nature of a compulsive world champion. Perhaps if she had done what we are now telling you to do, she would still be competing.

This Isn't Working

When it comes to weight training, it takes at least 6 weeks of consistent training to begin to notice physical changes in your body. That's 6 weeks of *consistent* training. Oftentimes people think they're training intensely when in fact they're pushing themselves while they lift but taking a ton of time between sets. In other words, be sure you're following our guidelines before you assume you're making little or no progress. However, if after 6 weeks of diligent gym work you don't notice a change—even if it's slight—you may consider tinkering with your routine. A few ways you may alter your routine are as follows:

◆ **Vary the number of reps.** Generally speaking, we like a range of 10 to 12, but that's not written in stone. Try decreasing the weight by 5 percent to 10 percent and bump up your rep range to 12 to 15.

◆ **Decrease the amount of rest between sets.** If you are resting for 2 minutes, decrease it to 1 minute. You'll probably have to decrease the weight by a few pounds, but you'll find it really challenging.

◆ **Change the exercises.** Most freeweight exercises we showed you have machine equivalents and vice versa. Try mixing it up for a while. Remember, the more you keep your muscles guessing, the better off you are.

To make gains in strength and in your appearance, you must continue to put stress on your muscles. If you are constantly doing sets of 10 reps with 10-pound biceps curls when you could clearly do an eleventh repetition, you're not going to see much of a change. Getting strong means using as many muscle fibers as possible during your exercise. The last few reps should be difficult. Once it becomes *easy,* you must increase the stress on the muscle by upping the weight you lift—that is, if you want to get stronger.

I'm Bored

No matter what the activity, weight training can get pretty boring if you're doing the same thing every time you hit the gym. Even if you increase the weight/reps or decrease your rest, if the basis of your routine is the same, you can become mentally tired. This is when you need to play around with some special techniques that can add a much-needed jolt to your program.

If you find that despite hard efforts, you don't appear to be getting stronger over the course of 3 to 4 weeks, it may be time for a rest or a change in your program. If you're exhibiting any of the signs of overtraining we outlined earlier, try taking a few extra days off. If you feel good but have just hit a plateau, you can try varying the program.

Changing a program every few months helps avoid mental boredom, but it also helps keep your muscles challenged. By varying the exercises from time to time, you ensure that you present new challenges for your muscles. Even the subtle change in angle from a freeweight exercise to its machine equivalent or switching from a barbell to dumbbells can give a muscle a little surprise and help push you through plateaus.

You can tinker with your exercise plan in countless ways. In the next few chapters, we show you some advanced techniques you can use to spice up your program.

The Least You Need to Know

◆ Now that you've learned the basics, it's time to assemble a solid routine.

◆ You can make tremendous gains in only 45 minutes a day.

◆ No matter how good your form, stiff and sore muscles are par for the course.

◆ Being enthusiastic is great; doing too much, too often can be bad.

◆ Changing your routine is great for your muscles and ensures you won't be bored.

In This Chapter

- ◆ Doin' it wrong
- ◆ Checking your ego at the door
- ◆ Slowing down

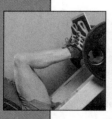
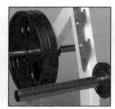
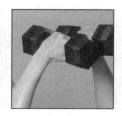
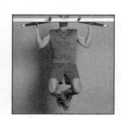
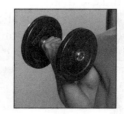
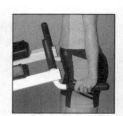

Chapter **14**

Don't Do It

After the last 13 chapters, you don't need to be a detective to figure out that we're fans of weight lifting. We like it for young and old, big and small, male and female. It's great for preventing injuries, improving sports performance, and helping you look good and feel better.

Still, lifting is not without some inherent dangers. Unfortunately, we see it all the time. Virtually every time we're in any gym—bare bones or high end—we see people doing things that make us cringe. Sometimes the culprit is form that clearly compromises the safety and effectiveness of the exercise. Other times it's the choice of exercise that bothers us.

In this chapter, we highlight some of the most common and egregious mistakes we see in the weight room. After all, the only thing worse than a workout that doesn't help you get any stronger is one that injures you.

I'll Take a Six-Pack

Next time you're at the gym, take a look around at all the people doing abdominal exercises. Maybe they're thinking that strong abdominal muscles help prevent lower back pain and injury or about how strengthening their abs will improve their game. More likely they're just thinking about how good their flat, athletic six-pack will look next time they walk down the beach. Regardless of the thought process, many of them are putting in lots and lots of effort and not getting much (except maybe a bad back) to show for their work. Why? Let's take a look at a couple of the most common mistakes well-intentioned but misguided lifters make.

Sit-Ups

Yes, sit-ups are a staple in high school gym classes, but although we're sure your phys-ed teacher was a swell guy, if he had you doing full sit-ups, he wasn't doing you any favors. (No, that doesn't excuse the spitballs you shot his way.) What's wrong with sit-ups? Nothing, except for two not-so-minor details: they're not safe, and they're not effective.

Here's why: when you anchor your feet (by having someone hold them down, placing them under a desk, or hooking them under a pad on an abdominal bench), the iliopsoas muscles in the front of your hips (along with other muscles, known as your hip flexors) help pull you up. If your hip flexors are working, it means your abdominal muscles aren't doing the lion's share of the work. In addition, by bringing those nasty hip flexors into the equation, you place undue stress on your lower back.

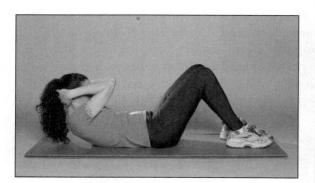

Full sit-ups aren't as safe or effective as crunches.

Flip back to Chapter 12 for the full rundown on good form for crunches, but here's a quick reminder: slowly curl forward for 3 seconds up to an angle of about 30°, pause, and slowly lower yourself back to the starting position. Be sure to keep your lower back pressed into the floor at all times, and keep your hands lightly clasped behind your head, with your elbows wide rather than tucked in front of you. Be sure to exhale on the way up and inhale on the return.

Double Leg Lifts with Straight Legs

The double leg lift is another classic gym move we wish would go the way of the pet rock. It's supposed to strengthen your lower abs, but it's really just an exercise in futility. What's wrong with leg lifts? Where do we start? Much like the full sit-up, this exercise doesn't work your abs effectively because your hip flexors produce the movement. Adding injury to insult, they place a tremendous stress on your lower back.

> **Weight a Minute**
>
> Exercises such as full sit-ups and straight-legged leg lifts are not only ineffective for strengthening your abdominal muscles, they're also dangerous for your lower back. Protect your back by keeping it pressed into the mat and not anchoring your feet when you do crunches.

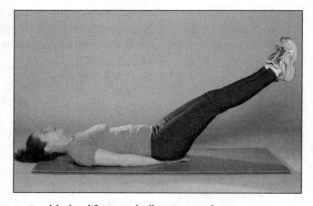

Double leg lifts are challenging and impressive—but ineffective.

A far better option is the reverse crunch we showed you in Chapter 12. Although far less impressive-looking than leg lifts, the reverse crunch is a safe way to work your lower abs. Keep the movement small, and keep your lower back pressed into the mat at all times.

Lift your tailbone a few inches off the floor, pause at the top, and slowly return to the starting position. Think about pulling your bellybutton down to the floor as you raise your legs.

Bad Bench

"How much do you bench?" The question is repeated around the gym as often as "Who are you wearing?" is at the Academy Awards. It's one of the questions we hate the most. Since Chapter 1, we've been stressing that the goal of lifting should be to gain strength, not to demonstrate strength, yet many lifters persist in the dangerous and counterproductive practice of "maxing out" on the bench press. Worse still, the form they use to help show off their "strength" generally ranges from poor to atrocious.

Here are the most common mistakes we see:

◆ Arching your back
◆ Holding your breath
◆ Lowering the bar too fast
◆ Bouncing the bar off your chest

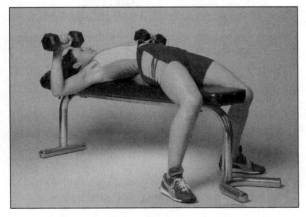

Cheating on the bench makes the lift much easier—and much more dangerous.

Sure, this makes it a lot easier to impress your friends, but all too often the result of bad bench press form is a shoulder, wrist, or back injury. These form faux pas keep Deidre's

physical therapy practice thriving but don't do much for the lifters who commit them.

Proper bench press form means keeping your knees bent and your feet flat on the floor at all times. If your back arches off the bench in this position, place your feet on the bench or use 45-pound plates as risers. Slowly lift and lower the bar—3 seconds in each direction; pause for a split second at your chest; never bounce the bar. Exhale on the way up, and inhale on the way down. Last but not least, always use a spotter. If one isn't available, use a machine or dumbbells.

Oh-No Bent Rows

In Chapter 8 we showed you dumbbell rows—a perfectly effective and safe way to strengthen the muscles of your middle and lower back. The only bad thing we can say about the dumbbell row is that you have to do the exercise with one arm at a time. Unfortunately, rather than using dumbbells for the exercise, many lifters use a barbell and take care of both sides of their body in one fell swoop. The problem is that while you're working out the muscles on both sides of your lower back, you're also compromising safety by bending forward. (In case you're brushing up for a biomechanics test, the technical term for this is unsupported forward flexion.) We're not suggesting you'll get hurt any and every time you bend forward at the waist, but we do question the wisdom of doing it that way when there's a safer alternative. By placing your knee and nonworking hand on the bench during the dumbbell version, you protect your lower back yet still get every bit as good a workout for the muscles in your back.

While we're being picky about back exercises, let's look at the physical therapist's best friend—an exercise known as the good morning. In the good morning, you place a barbell across your back, bend forward at the waist, and then return to an upright, standing position. The idea of the good morning is to strengthen your lower back—which it may do.

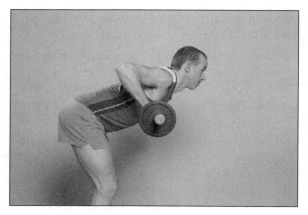

The barbell bent row is not nearly as safe as the dumbbell version.

Unfortunately, it also jeopardizes the structures of your lower back in the process.

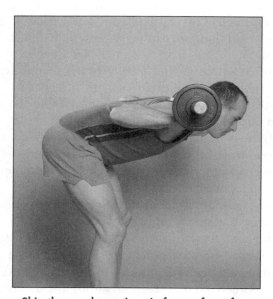

Skip the good mornings in favor of a safer alternative like the back raise.

Fortunately, there are exercises that are equally effective and far safer alternatives. Flip back to Chapter 8 and review the back raise we taught you. The 45° angle of the bench protects your lower back, yet you can still get a great workout. Just remember to raise your torso in a slow, controlled fashion rather than swinging and using momentum.

Which Way to the Beach?

If the bench press is the single most abused exercise in the weight room, the biceps curl is probably a close second. Bulging biceps look great, but just throwing a ton of weight on the bar and getting the bar up any way you can isn't the safest or most effective way to get those "big guns."

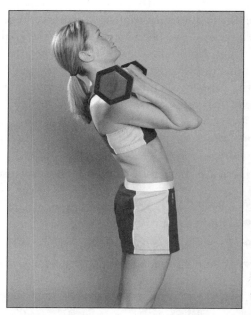

What's wrong with this picture? Try the arched back, raised elbows, and forward pelvis to start.

Once again, cheating makes it much easier to move more weight—it's just not doing your arms any good. Here are a few common but crucial mistakes you should avoid:

◆ Arching your back

◆ Holding your breath

◆ Throwing your pelvis forward

◆ Raising your elbows

◆ Moving the bar too fast

Keep your shoulders over your hips and your hips over your ankles. Don't let your elbows rise during the exercise—that involves your shoulders and does your biceps no good. Review the form we outlined in Chapter 11 for a full rundown.

Exploring Exploding

Throughout this book, we've advocated lifting with a 3-second up, 3-second down cadence. There's nothing magical about that pace, but we favor it because it's slow enough to minimize momentum, yet not so slow that keeping track of the timing becomes harder than the lift itself. Our main concern is that you lift in a slow, controlled fashion, so as to keep constant tension on the working muscle.

We'll spare you the physics lecture, but know this—by lifting fast, you put much more stress on your connective tissue and greatly increase your chance of injury. Furthermore, you bring momentum into the equation and make the exercise much easier, which is the exact opposite of what you want. When Deidre lifted competitively, her goal was to demonstrate strength by hoisting the most weight she could. To achieve her aim, she used every trick in the book to help move the bar. Lifting fast was one such trick. Now that she's no longer competing, her goals in the weight room are to stay strong and healthy. Because she doesn't really care how much weight she moves—only how strong she gets—she pays strict attention to technique. By adhering to the 3 seconds up, 3 seconds down cadence—with a slight pause in between—she ensures maximum results and minimum risk.

1,001, 1,002, 1,003 ...

Most of the horrors we've outlined so far are typically testosterone-fueled, but the ladies shouldn't be so quick to cast stones in the gym. What wrong could the fairer sex possibly do? Next time you're in the gym, let your eyes wander over to the abduction or adduction machines designed to strengthen the muscles of your outer and inner thighs. What you'll

most likely see is someone doing sets of 50 or 100 or more reps. That same strategy is why you see people doing hundreds of crunches. Why? Usually it's in a misguided attempt to "slim" and "tone" the area.

So what's the problem? That burning sensation you feel at the end of the set has absolutely nothing to do with burning fat in that area. If you work a muscle hard enough, it will grow, not shrink. If you choose a weight that lets you do that many reps, it's just a waste of time. There's not enough stimulus to cause any growth, but it's sure not going to make anything shrink. Think about it—those grunting guys off in the corner aren't doing those arm exercises in the hopes that their muscles will shrink!

Flex Facts

You can do crunches 'til the Cubs win the World Series and still not lose your gut. Weight training is certainly an important component in long-term weight control, but if your goal is trimming and toning your thighs or flattening your midsection, it's important not to neglect your cardiovascular exercise. It's still the fastest way to burn calories.

Hopefully this chapter will help you to avoid some of the most common pitfalls that snare even the best-intentioned lifters in the weight room. Remember that weight lifting is a means to an end—not an end unto itself. Keep your ego in check, focus on form, and lift away.

The Least You Need to Know

◆ Make each exercise as challenging as possible.
◆ Lifting more weight isn't always a good thing.
◆ Hundreds of reps are a waste of time.

In This Chapter

- ◆ Using SuperSlow and plyometrics
- ◆ Performing supersets
- ◆ Getting negative
- ◆ Lending a hand

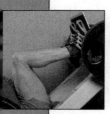
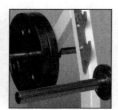
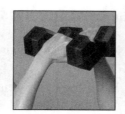
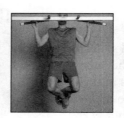
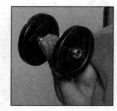
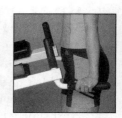

Chapter **15**

Getting Fancy

Like a good love affair, your initial foray in the gym will be filled with grand expectations and great enthusiasm. After a while, that puppy-love stage simmers down to a nice, solid routine—until at some point you need another spark of enthusiasm to keep you enthralled. People who keep plodding along with the same old routine are likely to experience gains in strength, but after a while, what we call the same-old-thing syndrome is likely to bring them to a grinding plateau, physically and mentally.

Like death and taxes, this familiarity-breeds-contempt syndrome happens to the best of us. Sometimes just taking a short break from the gym is enough to get you back into the swing of things; sometimes more drastic means are necessary.

To spice up your workout, we have detailed several techniques you can work into your routine. It seems too obvious to mention, but many people—especially newcomers to the gym—assume they need to do the same workout day after day, year after year. Nothing could be further from the truth. Initially, it's important that you learn how to perform the variety of exercises available to you. However, after you've built a solid base, one of the really fun and challenging aspects of weight training is designing new routines to improve your fitness. Think of training as a journey in which you're traveling on your own unique route. As fitness guru Steve Ilg says, "A fitness program is not punishment for an imperfect body, but a sign of care. Love your body as it is. Then act to keep it well suited to the life tasks to which you are called."

SuperSlow

The *SuperSlow* Protocol is an exercise technique developed in the early 1980s by Ken Hutchins. The basis of the technique is to perform a single repetition for 15 seconds: 10 seconds up and 5 seconds down. Because each repetition takes so long, a set may consist of only 3 to 5 repetitions. By slowing things down so much, momentum is all but eliminated and orthopedic stress is minimized. Of course, curious bystanders might think you've suffered a stroke. No matter; lifting like this requires great effort and powers of concentration.

Bar Talk

SuperSlow is a protocol that, as the name suggests, involves extremely slow movement—10 seconds for the positive phase and 5 seconds for the negative. SuperSlow is a very challenging but safe method of strength training.

SuperSlow definitely works, but many people find it tedious to adhere to this slow-mo approach. However, many SuperSlow devotees take a hard-line approach to their training, insisting that it is the only way to go. This, of course, is myopic and shouldn't concern you. What is relevant is that by moving faster in the eccentric or negative phase than in the concentric or positive phase, you reduce the amount of recovery for the concentric phase. (Unless we overload with accentuated negatives, the value of moving slowly during the negatives is questionable.) Finally, although the 10-5 speed accomplishes what it says—limiting momentum and orthopedic stress while keeping muscular tension high—the 10-5 speed is not the only option. Movement cadences of 5-10, 10-10, 3-1-3, or other combinations that minimize momentum may be just as effective.

Let's consider the advantages of the SuperSlow system:

◆ You will get stronger.

◆ No momentum to propel the weight.

◆ You risk no orthopedic injuries from using too much weight.

◆ It's safe.

Now consider the disadvantages:

◆ Because the technique is so slow and the weight is so much lighter, some people may be turned off of using it.

◆ You have to pay attention to how long each repetition is by using a clock with a second hand, metronome, or timer. Unless you work with a partner, your concentration is split between counting and lifting.

Having warned you about the boredom factor, we certainly think SuperSlow is worth trying. It is demanding, but when you get into it, you'll find that the focused concentration required brings a new energy your workout may be sorely lacking. No, we're not in agreement with the SuperSlow people who claim it's the only way to lift. Nor do we agree that you need to do all your workouts that way. But if you're looking for a new workout wrinkle, it's a fine way to increase the intensity of some of your workouts.

Flex Facts

Although Dr. Wayne Westcott has found that SuperSlow can be an effective means of making strength gains, participants in the training program reported that they found the method particularly tedious. Having a riotous good time isn't necessarily the goal of a weight-lifting program, but odds are you have a better chance of sticking with it if it's enjoyable.

Plyometrics: Not So Fast

In the days of the Berlin Wall, East German athletes supposedly gained some of their potent athleticism from a funky method of training known as *plyometrics*. Since that dreaded wall has crumbled, this dynamic method of strength training has gained considerable popularity. So what in the name of Uta Pippig is plyometrics?

Basically, it's exercises that emphasize bounding and explosive movements. In theory, doing exercises that emphasize a particular movement, say jumping on and off a platform as quickly as possible, will elicit great gains when you ask your body to perform the less-exaggerated version. According to advocates of plyometrics, this type of training helps build explosive power, jumping ability, and quickness.

Bar Talk

Plyometrics is a method of strength training that involves bounding and jumping exercises. Both the safety and effectiveness of plyometrics are questionable, and we caution against the use of most plyometric exercises.

Let's take a look at what's behind this hop, skip, and jump craze. Plyometrics attempts to take advantage of the elasticity of the muscle by prestretching it before contraction. In other words, plyometrics uses your body's natural defense mechanisms to help produce a more forceful muscle action.

Let us explain. We told you about muscle spindles, the sensors in your muscles that respond to excessive stretching in an attempt to protect the muscles. As you may recall, when you stretch too far or too fast, muscle spindles try to contract the muscle before it gets injured or overstretched. Plyometric exercises intentionally and forcefully prestretch the muscle. This means the muscle spindles are excited, and that helps lead to a more forceful contraction.

Here's an example of how it works: assuming you're sitting right now, stand up and jump as high as you can. If you're like the rest of us, you probably bent down into a coiled position just before you jumped. That's prestretching the muscle. You do the same kind of thing before swinging a baseball bat or kicking a soccer ball.

Common plyometrics exercises include throwing a medicine ball (a soft, weighted ball), as well as a variety of difficult drills in which you jump, hop, or bound—often off of or over boxes. Sounds good, and it is if you can ward off injuries. However, we have some serious concerns about the effectiveness, and more important, the safety, of plyometrics for both beginners and elite athletes.

When doing plyometric exercises, you place significant stress on your musculoskeletal system, especially when using added weight such as a bar or a weighted vest, or when jumping from a platform. Even if the risk of injury is acceptable—and we don't think it is—there is little evidence that plyometrics are worth the risk.

When executing a plyometric movement, you often do not work the muscle through a full range of motion (ROM). Even if you do, although there is tremendous tension on the muscle at the beginning of the movement, the momentum produced by the fast speed of the movement decreases muscle tension throughout most of the ROM.

Weight a Minute

Plyometrics place tremendous stress on your joints and connective tissue. Because of the danger and the fact that more conventional methods are at least as effective, plyometrics should only be done by advanced athletes—if at all.

Having said that, many fitness experts swear by plyometrics. And the number of world-class athletes who use these techniques is too large to mention. The important thing to keep in mind if you're going to try some of these exercises is to be sure your technique is impeccable, and always do a thorough warm-up. Hopping around like a kangaroo on speed when you're cold is a certain way to court injury.

Here are the advantages of plyometric training:

◆ Minimal equipment requirements

◆ Some simpler exercises may benefit agility

And for the disadvantages of plyometric training:

◆ High potential for injury to connective tissue (tendons and ligaments)

◆ Risk of hip, knee, and ankle strains and sprains

◆ Danger of stress fractures

Earlier we mentioned that plyometrics have gained considerable attention in the past few years. As we said, some experts swear by them; some swear against them. Even though the all-pro wide receiver for your favorite football team says doing plyometrics has added 2 inches to his vertical leap, it's safe to assume he could jump a lot higher than most mere mortals before he started bounding off of boxes. Elite athletes sometimes reach elite status despite their training rather than because of it.

In 1985, the New York Giants used plyometrics extensively in their training en route to winning the Super Bowl. That year advocates of explosive movements were in their glory, pointing to the Giants as an example of the superiority of plyometrics over conventional strength-training methods. The wrinkle in the equation came the next year when the Washington Redskins won the whole enchilada. You see, Dan Riley, the strength and conditioning coach for the Redskins and one of the most respected men in the business, is an outspoken critic of plyometrics. Under Riley's watchful eye, the Redskins use only slow, controlled movements in the weight room because he sees no reason to jeopardize the safety of his multimillion-dollar players.

Would these same teams have won if they had traded strength coaches? Who knows? The bottom line is that anecdotal evidence supplied by individuals, even great ones, does not mean you

should follow their training plans. For every story of an athlete who excels using plyometrics, there's another who does just as well with safer methods, or worse, one who got hurt using plyometrics.

Certain simple agility drills such as a football player running through tires or even rope-jumping can be classified as low-level plyometric exercises, and we'd be hard-pressed to argue against them as a means of improving skill and dexterity. Still, due to the increased risk of injury as well as the lack of proof that most plyometric exercises are more effective than conventional means of strength training, it seems that they should be used with extreme caution, if at all.

Supersets

Now here's a technique we really like. *Supersets* are an advanced technique that involves performing two different exercises with little rest in between.

Bar Talk

Supersets are an advanced strength-training method that involves doing two exercises with no rest in between. The most common way to superset is to do exercises that stress the same muscles, but in some cases you work opposing muscles in succession.

Sometimes you work opposing muscle groups without rest, for example, a biceps curl immediately followed by a triceps extension. The more common method is to do a set of a single-joint movement like a bench flye, which isolates your pecs, and then go right into a bench press without any rest. By prefatiguing your pecs with the flye, you have made the bench press more challenging. Why? Normally, when you do a hard set on the bench press, your triceps, which straighten your elbow, are prone to tiring out before you've fully exhausted your pecs. However, during the flye, your triceps don't do any work; your pecs do. When you then move to the bench press, your pecs get an extra-hard workout without worrying about the tri's being the weak link.

To effectively perform a superset, you must be sure you have access to each machine or bench you'll be using. For instance, if you want to get a good shoulder workout, you might do a lateral raise right before a shoulder press. However, before starting either, you'll need to have a light set of dumbbells for the lateral raises and a heavier set waiting for you for the presses. Any time lost fumbling around on a rack for the weights takes away from the effectiveness of the exercise. This doesn't mean you should race around between sets, but it is important to segue from one to the other as smoothly and efficiently as possible. Another thing to keep in mind is that because your muscle is prefatigued before the second exercise, you'll need to decrease the weight you use by about 25 percent.

Because supersets are so demanding, we don't advocate using them too often. Rather, it's a way to tweak your routine when it gets stale or when you're unable to make any progress in the strength department. When Jonathan worked as a personal trainer, he liked to surprise his clients every 2 weeks or so by throwing in one superset per body part. Often they grumbled and groaned because it required extra effort to combat the prefatigued muscles. However, the clients who really wanted to make progress enjoyed the extra challenge.

Remember, though, that supersets should be used judiciously. Done too often, you run the risk of overdoing it. In Chapter 16, we give you more examples of specific ways to use supersets in your workouts.

Here are the advantages of superset training:

◆ It saves time.

◆ It allows extra focus on certain muscles.

And the disadvantages of superset training:

◆ You may not be able to use the machine you want immediately if someone else is on it.

◆ You run the risk of overtraining.

Be Negative

No, we aren't suggesting that you develop a lousy attitude. We mean do *negatives*. The negative portion of the exercise is the lowering phase of the exercise. Physiologically, you can lower about 40 percent more weight than you can lift. In the course of a normal set, you're obviously lifting and lowering the same amount of weight, but there are ways to add extra stress to the negative.

Bar Talk

Negatives are an advanced technique in which you stress the negative or eccentric phase of an exercise. They're a great way to get your body acclimated to a new weight when you've reached a strength plateau.

When you stress the negative phase, you also increase the amount of delayed onset muscle soreness that can occur, so it must be used judiciously and in a controlled manner.

Negatives are a great way to get used to handling a little extra weight and help push you through a plateau. When Deidre first started competing, her bench press was stuck at 135 pounds for an eternity. Not bad for a 122-pound woman, but still not good enough if she wanted to beat the best. To get her acclimated to the extra weight, her coach had her do negatives with 145 pounds for a couple workouts. Before you could say *pectoralis major*, she was benching up a storm. (For the record, Deidre's best bench press in competition is 176 pounds.)

You can do two types of negative work:

◆ The first requires a spotter who will lift the weight and stand by as you slowly lower it— no faster than a 3-second count on the way down. Do each rep like this until you have completed your set. Even though your muscles can handle an extra 40 percent for this type of training, you should start out with only 15 to 20 percent above your normal training weight. Because you're using more weight than you can move on your own, a trusted spotter is crucial, especially if you're doing a freeweight exercise.

◆ The second type involves body-weight exercises such as pull-ups and dips. If your gym doesn't have an assisted chin/dip machine, negatives are a good way to work up to full-body-weight chins and dips. Use a small platform to bring yourself to the top position for either of these exercises, step off the platform, and slowly lower yourself. Repeat this for a set of 10 or 12 or until you can no longer control the speed of the movement.

Spot Me

Here's a tip to keep in mind when you try negatives: rather than thinking of lowering the weight, focus on resisting it, as if you were still trying to lift it. For instance, if you're using 15-pound dumbbells, think of pushing up with 14 pounds worth of force. This way the weight will slowly overcome your effort, and you'll be sure to move nice and slowly.

The following are advantages of negatives:

◆ Good strength gains
◆ Helps you break through plateaus

The following are disadvantages of negatives:

◆ Need a spotter for most of the exercises
◆ Possibility of increased muscle soreness

Breakdowns

Breakdown training is another high-intensity technique we highly endorse. Breakdowns require reducing the amount of resistance at the point when you reach muscular failure. Usually, a 20 percent decrease in resistance will allow you to eke out 3 to 4 additional repetitions.

Bar Talk

With **breakdowns,** once you fatigue, you decrease the weight being used and do a few extra reps. This method allows you to reach failure twice on the same set and may promote even better strength gains than more conventional techniques.

For example, let's say you're bench pressing 75 pounds 10 times. When you try another rep, your muscles resist and the spotter has to help you with the lift. At that point, the spotter strips the bar down to 60 pounds, and you then try to squeeze out another 3 or 4 reps. If you're really ambitious, you can strip the bar down to 50 pounds and try for 2 or 3 more reps. Try not to exceed 15 or 16 reps for the total set.

Breakdowns using a bar require a spotter, but when doing dumbbell exercises, all you have to do is have an extra pair waiting for you when you reach failure with the original weight. It's an even smoother transition when using a machine; all you have to do is move the pin to a lighter weight and get back to work.

The following are advantages of breakdown training:

◆ It's a great wake-up call to stalled muscle/ strength gains.
◆ When using machines, you can work extra hard without the need of a spotter.
◆ Your workout will become more aerobic because your heart rate will be doing the conga.
◆ It builds concentration and mental tenacity.

And a disadvantage of breakdown training:

◆ Spotters are needed for most freeweight exercises.

Help Me

Assisted training—a fancy name for having a spotter help you push out a few more reps—is similar to breakdown training in the sense that it allows you to do a few extra repetitions after you have reached failure. In assisted training, rather than decreasing the resistance by stripping the bar, switching dumbbells, or moving the pin, your spotter helps you to do 2 to 4 extra reps.

The key to successful assisted training is a good spotter. To get the most effective bang for your buck, you need a spotter who helps you along just enough but not so much as to make the extra repetitions useless. As the lifter, your job is to do your best to keep the weight moving. This requires maximum effort as well as good concentration. In addition to allowing you to do a few extra positive reps, assisted training gives you a great workout in the negative phase. This means you control the weight on the way down to the count of 4. On the negative phase, the spotter merely is there so you don't drop the bar on your head.

Don't overdo assisted reps. If you try for more than 4 post-fatigue reps, you're likely to give your spotter a great workout, because it's doubtful you'll have anything left in the tank. Again, the key thing to keep in mind when you're lifting is to push to momentary failure without compromising technique. Remember: form, form, form.

The following are advantages of assisted training:

◆ It's a great way to work harder than usual.

◆ It stresses negative phase.

◆ You don't need to switch equipment or change weights.

◆ It's a good way to offer and receive encouragement from your fellow lifters.

And one disadvantage of assisted training:

◆ It requires a good spotter.

Any of the methods we've described are well suited to jump-starting your training if you've found yourself in a bit of a rut. Regardless of which of these techniques you employ, pay careful attention to form, and remember that you'll need extra recovery time after any of these workouts. That's why we keep stressing that you don't try to use them too often. However, when you find yourself in a rut, any of these techniques are a great way to break through.

The Least You Need to Know

◆ When you find yourself stuck on a physical or mental plateau, it's time to vary your routine.

◆ SuperSlow is a protocol that, as the name suggests, involves extremely slow movement—10 seconds for the positive phase and 5 seconds for the negative.

◆ Plyometrics is a method of strength training that involves bounding and jumping exercises.

◆ Supersets is an advanced strength-training method that involves doing two exercises with no rest between.

◆ Negatives is an advanced technique in which you stress the negative or eccentric phase of an exercise.

◆ Advanced training techniques are excellent, but beware—they're difficult and shouldn't be overused.

In This Chapter

◆ Training like a caveman

◆ Pushing versus pulling

◆ Working your upper and lower body

◆ Performing supersets and circuit training

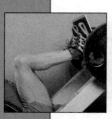
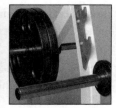
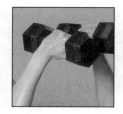
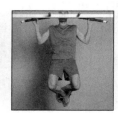
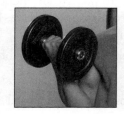
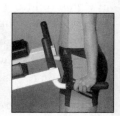

Chapter 16

High Tech

In the August 1999 issue of *Men's Health* magazine, Chris Ballard wrote an amusing article about how your average caveman was as fit as today's Olympic athlete. Goofy, yes, but quirky enough to consider. To survive, your handy primitive had to have the endurance of a marathon runner to track game and a sprinter's speed to close in on a tiring elk. In the normal course of a day, a caveman lifted stones and tree trunks the way your typical NFL lineman pumps iron. Okay, his posture and table manners left something to be desired, but the point remains that his lofty feats of strength and endurance stemmed from the endless variety of ever-changing physical demands required of him.

Despite our fast-paced, sophisticated lives, we are physical beings genetically programmed to do vigorous exercise. Lifting weights is a modern means of filling this need. But if you stick to the same old routine week after week, you are likely to get bored.

The willingness to change your routine regularly will not only keep you mentally challenged, but will ensure that your body adapts to the new stress as well. Meeting these constantly changing demands will help push you to a higher level of fitness. In this chapter, we give you a variety of examples of how to use some of the techniques we described in Chapter 15.

Each is more physically challenging than the basic training we've described up until now, and each will have added benefits. They're not techniques you need to try early on in your lifting life, but they may come in handy if you want to give your workouts some extra *oomph* or if you ever have to flee from a woolly mammoth.

Split Routines

Although we generally prefer that you work all your muscles on the same day, it's not the only way to go. Many strength experts like to use a *split routine*. These routines combine muscle groups or body parts to be worked out on alternating days. For example, on Monday you may work your chest, shoulders, and triceps; Tuesday, back and biceps; and Wednesday, legs and abs. When you're doing a fairly high volume of exercises, split routines enable you to avoid spending all day in the gym. And because you're not working your entire body, you're able to do more exercises per body part as well as work out more intensely. The more focus you bring to your workout, the better.

 Bar Talk

A **split routine** is a regimen in which you divide your workout over 2 (or more) days. Split routines are particularly useful if you want to do more than two or three exercises per body part.

In a split routine, you usually work each body part twice per week. The key to a successful split is to avoid using the same muscles on consecutive days. So if you did a chest/shoulders/triceps workout on Monday, you'd let those body parts recover until Wednesday or Thursday.

The beginning routines we described for you in Chapter 13 include about 15 exercises that should take you about 45 minutes—a manageable load for your mind and body. You can add a few extra exercises and still be able to finish in less than an hour. However, if you want to get stronger faster or refine the look of your body, doing multiple exercises for each body part is probably the way to go. If you find yourself upping the number of exercises you're doing on any one day (say 20 or more), it's probably time to think about a split routine.

The following are advantages to a split routine:

◆ It allows you to incorporate more exercises than in a full-body routine.

◆ It lets you place more focus on specific body parts.

◆ If it's done correctly, you'll get stronger faster.

And some disadvantages of a split routine:

◆ It requires more days per week in the gym.

◆ It allows fewer rest/recovery days.

Okay, let's assume you're a split-routine kind of person. Let's look at some of the best split routines.

Push-Pull

One popular and logical way to break up your exercises for a split routine is the push-pull split. Pushing exercises are those such as the bench press or military press, where the resistance is moved away from your body during the positive phase. Pulling exercises such as rowing and pull-downs bring the resistance toward the body. Pushing exercises stress the muscles of your chest, shoulders, and triceps. Pulling movements work your back muscles and biceps. The key feature of the push-pull split routine, or any other good split, is that the same muscles are not stressed on consecutive days. If you do use them consecutive days, you don't allow your muscles enough recovery time, and they're too weak to do the job.

The push-pull split routine refers to working all muscle groups that push on one day followed by working all muscles that pull on the other day. For example …

Monday/Thursday	Tuesday/Friday
Legs	Chest
Back	Shoulders
Biceps	Triceps

For the sake of balance, we've included all leg exercises on the pull day. Following is a solid sample routine using the push-pull split. This routine is probably our favorite way to split things up; it allows a nice balance between muscle groups and works well for most people.

Days 1 and 4

Body Part	Exercises
Legs	Leg press
	Leg extension
	Leg curl
	Standing calf raise
	Seated calf raise
Back	Lat pull-down
	Machine row
	Upright row
	Back extension
Biceps	Seated biceps curl
	Concentration curl
Abs	Reverse crunch
	Crunch
	Oblique crunch

Days 2 and 5

Body Part	Exercises
Chest	Bench press
	Incline press
	Decline press
	Dips
	Pec deck
Shoulders	Shoulder press
	Front raise
	Reverse flye
Triceps	Triceps pushdown
	Triceps kickback

This configuration groups the pushing exercises, like all the pressing movements, and keeps the pulling exercises together. The advantage the split routine offers is that all the muscles performing a similar routine are getting a good workout throughout the entire routine. When you work your pecs as in a bench press, you are also working your deltoids and your triceps. Move on to the shoulder press, and you're using your deltoids and triceps again. When you do a typical back exercise like a lat pull-down, your biceps are also doing a lot of work.

Upper-Lower

The upper-lower split routine is basically exactly what it says: upper body one day, lower body the next. Once again, it avoids using the same muscles on consecutive days. The upper-lower body split is especially effective if you want to emphasize your legs. On your lower body day, you get to concentrate heavily on your legs without worrying about having energy left for other body parts. Here's a sample program:

Monday/Thursday	Tuesday/Friday
Chest	Legs
Back	Abs
Shoulders	Lower back
Biceps	
Triceps	

Days 1 and 4

Body Part	Exercises
Legs	Leg press
	Leg extension
	Leg curl
	Standing calf raise
	Seated calf raise

continues

Days 1 and 4 (continued)

Body Part	Exercises
	Abduction
	Adduction
Abs	Reverse crunch
	Crunch
	Oblique crunch
Lower back	Back extension

Days 2 and 5

Body Part	Exercises
Back	Lat pull-down
	Machine row
	Upright row
Chest	Bench press
	Incline press
	Decline press
Shoulders	Military press
	Lateral raise
Biceps	Seated biceps curl
	Concentration curl
Triceps	Triceps pushdown
	Triceps kickback

A split routine makes sense if you're doing a lot of sets or, say, training for a power-oriented sport such as football. Trying to do too much in one day is bound to lead to a lack of concentration and enthusiasm. Breaking up your routine allows your muscles ample recovery time between workouts, but keep in mind that your body recovers as a unit, not just as individual muscles. A split routine guarantees you'll be in the gym on consecutive days during the week, which puts an extra demand on your body. It's wise to eat well and get plenty of rest no matter how hard you work out, but once you start training, more rest and nutrition becomes even more important.

Often, the drive that prompts people to go to a split routine is the same impulse that leads to chronic fatigue. Recognizing the signs of overtraining—irritability, sleeplessness, loss of appetite, and so on—before you smack into the dreaded wall is key if you hope to stay healthy.

Superset Routines

In Chapter 15, we told you that a superset is a pair of exercises performed with no rest in between. (Again, you can superset opposing muscle groups or the same muscle groups.) We also told you that we really like supersets as a way of pushing your muscles real hard.

Now let's look at superset routines for the same muscle groups. One of the best reasons for performing supersets is that you can get an extremely effective workout without the increased risk of orthopedic injuries from using too much weight. In fact, because your muscles are taxed harder, you usually use less weight when doing a superset.

Spot Me

We love supersets, but they need to be used judiciously. Don't try supersets more than once a week, and be conservative when selecting the weight for your exercises. The key to a successful superset is prefatiguing the muscle—so don't hold back on the first set.

Yes, it's an ego-buster if you get hung up on how much is *enough*, but unless you decrease the weight for the second set by about 25 percent, you'll never manage to do more than a couple reps on the second exercise.

The first time Jonathan tried doing a superset years ago, he did a good hard set of flyes to exhaust his pecs and jumped right to a bench press. Ambitious lad that he was, his plan was to use the same amount for the bench press as he usually did. Halfway through his first rep, painful visions of a mouse in a trap came to mind. He struggled to finish one rep with his normal weight, checked his ego at the door, and graphically learned how effective pre-exhaustion can be.

Nice Legs

As we mentioned in Chapter 7, squats and/or leg presses are the key exercises for most leg routines. One of the major pluses of either exercise is the fact that they work lots of large muscles in one shot: glutes, hamstrings, and quads. This is generally considered a positive, but the exercises don't allow you to place specific emphasis on one particular part of your legs. Supersets are a great tool to selectively stress a certain muscle of your legs.

A good quad superset routine requires that you have immediate access to whatever machines you'll be using in your routine. Because compound leg movements such as the squat or lunge work both your quadriceps and your hamstrings, doing a set of leg curls (hamstrings) or leg extensions (quads) before one of those exercises lets you choose which muscle you want to emphasize. Remember, moving from one routine to the other without rest means you'll need to decrease the weight of the second exercise by about 25 percent.

> **Quad Supersets**
> Leg extension/leg press
> *or*
> Leg extension/squat
> *or*
> Leg extension/lunge

Of the three, we prefer the first combination because the leg press enables you to work hard without the same safety concerns of a squat. If

you choose the squat, be sure to use a spotter, and be conservative with the weight. Lunges are a distant third place for our favorite quad superset combinations because you only use one leg at a time. Because the idea of a superset is to prefatigue the muscle and work it while it's tired, the rest you get between working each of your legs reduces the desired effect of the exercise.

> **Hamstring Supersets**
> Leg curls/leg press
> *or*
> Leg curls/squats
> *or*
> Leg curls/lunges

By throwing in a hamstring exercise before the compound movement, you shift the emphasis of the squat, leg press, or lunge to your hamstrings rather than your quads. Again, we prefer to use the leg press as the second exercise, but the others can work if necessary. (In Chapter 5, we told you that the primary function of the hamstrings is to bend your knees. This is true, but they also work in conjunction with the glutes to extend, or straighten, your hips as in the squat, leg press, or lunge.)

Just about everybody, from mountain bikers to senior citizens, can benefit from strong legs. Put simply: supersets are a guaranteed way to improve your leg strength.

Nice Pecs

Because most chest exercises also involve the smaller and weaker muscles of the shoulders and triceps, the chest is the perfect body part for supersetting. This will ensure that your pecs get a good workout without worrying about smaller muscles cutting your workout short. Although the bench press is often considered the single best pec exercise—and it is a very good one—your triceps, which are smaller and weaker than your pecs, are more likely to give out before your pecs. By prefatiguing your pecs in the first part of a superset, they get that extra oomph that will pay obvious dividends.

Pectoral Supersets

Dumbbell flyes/bench press or dumbbell press

or

Dumbbell flyes/chest press machine

or

Pec deck/chest press machine

Any of these options will do the trick nicely and really overload your pecs. The key to a successful pec superset is to be sure you really burn them out with the isolation exercise (pec deck or flyes) before moving on to the pressing exercise. Many experienced lifters complain that although they've gotten stronger and their arms have gotten bigger, the cosmetic changes in their pecs lag behind. That's usually due to an overdependence on pressing movements, where your triceps give out before your pecs are fully used. Supersets may be just the trick for such people.

Nice Delts

The deltoids respond nicely to a superset routine. The muscles are small enough that you don't have to use significant weight, especially when using this technique. As with other supersets, the key is to work as hard as possible on the first set. Done properly, your delts will be well on their way to exhaustion before you even begin the second set.

Deltoid Supersets

Lateral raises/military press

or

Lateral raises/shoulder press machine

or

Lateral raise machine/shoulder press machine

Again, the pattern is an isolation exercise followed by a compound movement. Don't plan on hailing a cab, fanning a campfire, or waving to a friend soon after a good deltoid superset—your shoulders should be too tired to raise your arms.

Nice Lats

Because the lats are so large, they tend to be very strong. Because they're so strong, the biceps are usually the weak link in an exercise like a lat pull-down or a chin-up. Without a machine such as the Nautilus Super Pullover, it's hard to isolate your lats. Unfortunately, this great machine has become a rarity in most gyms. (The Super Pullover was the first machine sold by Nautilus inventor Arthur Jones.) In its absence, the reverse flye is a decent way to prefatigue the muscles of your back, as well as your rear deltoids.

Lat/Rear Deltoid Supersets

Reverse flyes/cable rows

or

Reverse flyes/bent rows

Nice Traps

Supersets are also an excellent way to strengthen and fill out your traps. The best way to isolate them is with shrugs, so we include those. As we mentioned in Chapter 8, upright rows are a great exercise that work your deltoids and biceps in addition to your traps.

To place the concentration on your traps, prefatigue them with shrugs followed immediately by upright rows. Strong traps are essential for everything from carrying shopping bags to rowing.

Trap Superset

Shrugs/upright rows

Although we prefer prefatigue supersets to those that work opposing muscle groups, the latter is a good way to speed up a workout on days when you're pressed for time.

Following is an example of exercises you can put back to back. In each case, the movement is in the same plane—what varies is the direction of the resistance. For instance, a lat pull-down and a military press are essentially the same movement. In one case (military press) the resistance is pushing you down and in the other (lat pull-down) it's pulling you up.

Here are a few examples of opposing supersets:

◆ Leg extensions/leg curls

◆ Abduction/adduction

◆ Lat pull-downs/shoulder presses

◆ Machine rows/chest press machine or bench presses

◆ Upright rows/dips

◆ Crunches/back extensions

Circuit City

Circuit training is defined as a series of resistance exercises performed one after the other with minimal rest between exercises. By *minimal* we mean approximately 30 seconds or less. This fast-paced, aerobically based routine has also become increasingly popular in class settings. Many fitness experts consider circuit training a compromise between strength training and cardiovascular exercise. Strictly speaking, it is; however, it's a good compromise. So although you're neither maximizing your muscular payoff nor getting as good a cardiovascular workout as you would if you went for a run in the park, you are building strength and burning calories.

In circuit training, the amount of weight you use is considerably less than you would normally use—usually 40 percent to 60 percent of your usual weight for the same exercise. One of the advantages to this type of training is that it can increase local muscular endurance due to the low rest period between exercises. Another advantage is that it saves significant time, making it ideal for people who have limited time to commit to the gym.

Here's our take on circuit training: the continuous, or near continuous, activity of circuit training does raise your heart rate, leading some to believe that your cardiovascular system will benefit from such exercise. The problem with this reasoning is that the physiology behind raising your heart rate while lifting is different during traditional cardiovascular training such as jogging, cycling, and swimming.

Why? Follow this short physiology lesson: when you run, swim, or bike, your heart rate quickens, as does the amount of blood your heart pumps with each beat. On the other hand, when you lift, your heart rate increases, but the volume of blood pumped with each beat remains about the same and sometimes actually decreases. The point of the lesson? An elevated heart rate is not always an indicator that your heart is getting stronger. If that were the case, you could start a fitness movement by telling people to shelve their running shoes and bicycles and replace those workouts with a steady diet of scary movies. I can hear the infomercial now: "Hey man, how'd you run such a good marathon? Hill work?" "No, *Silence of the Lambs!*" "You?" "*Halloween, Part 5!*"

The bottom line on circuit training is that although it may be a compromise between traditional strength and cardiovascular exercise, it's not nearly as effective as either one separately. Still, done from time to time, it can be another effective way to add pizzazz to your gym time.

The Least You Need to Know

◆ Diversifying your routine challenges your mind and body.

◆ The split routine is a way to train each body part more intensely.

◆ Supersets are a super way to bump up the intensity.

◆ Circuit training gives you some cardiovascular benefits along with strength gains.

In This Chapter

- ◆ Getting serious
- ◆ Sculpting away
- ◆ Grunting for power
- ◆ Going for the gold

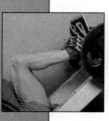
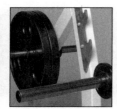
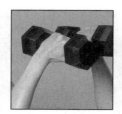
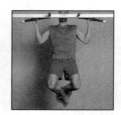
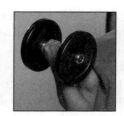
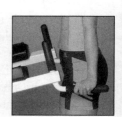

Chapter 17

And the Winner Is ...

The competitive aspect of strength training is a relatively esoteric part of the sports tapestry in this country. (Okay, try to name one Olympic weight lifter, powerlifter, or Mr. Olympia in the last 3 years.) However, knowing about the folks who are pushing the proverbial pedal to the metal can be both inspiring and just plain interesting. The relatively obscure competitive outlets available to weight lifters who just can't get enough of a good thing are bodybuilding, powerlifting, and Olympic weight lifting. Despite the immense differences found in these sports, each requires tremendous strength, technique, and discipline.

Most of you probably feel no need to compete. And many of the techniques employed by athletes in these disciplines contradict much of what we've taught you so far. Before this chapter, we've stressed that your goal in the weight room is to get as strong as possible and not show off for those around you. Well, guess what? Competitive lifters are the exception to the rule—for them, showing off is what it's all about.

Sometimes, challenging yourself to enter one of these contests will be the added incentive you need to push you to achieve a personal goal. But even if you have no interest in competing, it is interesting and informative to see how the muscleheads live.

Here's more than a bit about the rudiments of each sport.

Arnold's World

Who isn't familiar with Arnold Schwarzenegger, the six-time Mr. Olympia–turned-movie-mogul-turned-governor? In his prime, the Austrian Oak was one of the most imposing and muscular humans (at least we think he's human) to walk the planet. He certainly is the most well-known bodybuilder to ever strike a pose and was as instrumental as anyone in popularizing this oft-misunderstood sport. Arnold had some help, however, from legends of the sport such as Franco Colombo, Frank Zane, Lou Ferrigno, and Lee Haney, to name a few.

What made Schwarzenegger so popular? Aside from his enormous personality, his physique was extraordinary. At 6 feet 2 inches and 235 pounds, his measurements were the stuff sculptors pine for:

> **Arms:** 22 inches
>
> **Chest:** 57 inches
>
> **Waist:** 34 inches
>
> **Thighs:** 28.5 inches
>
> **Calves:** 20 inches

It's very difficult for a man of that height to pack on that much muscularity while remaining so exquisitely proportioned. Typically, bodybuilders who are densely muscled and symmetrically proportioned tend to be shorter, because it is easier for a smaller frame to give the appearance of greater muscle mass. In fact, one of Arnold's chief rivals during his heyday was Franco Columbo, a man so strong he was able to blow up a hot water bottle like a balloon until it exploded. This Italian dynamo had similar measurements, but he was nearly a foot shorter. Because Arnold was so statuesque, he won easily.

To excel at bodybuilding, one needs to have an incredible work ethic as well as an extraordinary genetic predisposition toward muscular growth. Simply put, without Mom and Dad's generous DNA, Arnold might still be in Austria doing who knows what. (He certainly would not be married to a Kennedy and one of the richest men in Hollywood—not that there's anything wrong with that.) A strong work ethic and favorable genetics are prerequisites for hitting the big time, but there's plenty of room in the sport for regular (lesser) oaks like you and me.

The goal of the sport is simple: to sculpt your body, giving it as much size and definition as possible. Perhaps more than any other sport, in bodybuilding diet is given as much attention as training, especially near competition time. Why? People can win or lose based upon whether or not they were on target with their diets.

A typical bodybuilding routine consists of 3 to 6 sets of 12 to 15 repetitions. Rest in between sets is usually no more than 60 to 90 seconds. Many of the advanced techniques we wrote about in Chapters 13 and 15—supersets, breakdowns, pre-exhaustion, and negatives—are standard fare here to achieve maximum results.

Due to the high volume of exercises and short rest sets used, bodybuilders cause an increase in muscle size through hypertrophy of existing muscle fibers. Muscle enlargement may also be attributed to an increase in capillaries, the smallest blood vessels. It appears that an increase in capillaries is associated with the high intensity and higher volume of strength training common among bodybuilders but not found in powerlifters and Olympic weight lifters.

Weight a Minute

Strength training increases the size and strength of not only muscle tissue, but of tendons and ligaments as well. Without this adaptation, damage to ligaments and tendons would be more likely to occur. The use (or abuse) of steroids, which unfortunately is common among professional bodybuilders, causes rapid increases in size and strength of skeletal tissue without the requisite strength in tendons and ligaments. As a result, tendon tears are common in athletes who abuse steroids.

Competition Anyone?

A bodybuilding contest is a little like a Miss America pageant. Although instead of the swimsuit and evening gown parade, athletes clad in little more than a cocktail napkin display their physical wares. The show itself consists of two phases: prejudging and the actual competition. Prejudging, which takes place first, is the weeding-out process. Competitors are lined up and instructed to strike several standard poses. The competitors who cut the mustard are asked to come back to go head-to-head during the next phase. The prime-time event has participants in light-, middle-, and heavyweight classes.

Each competitor performs a 5-minute routine he feels highlights his physique. After each competitor has performed his individual routine, they all come out for a face-off or pose-down, which consists of freestyle posing. With the bright lights blazing and music blaring, it's rather a surreal scene. Judges choose the winner using a point system based on muscle size, definition, symmetry, and the skill demonstrated during the posing routine.

While men's bodybuilding has been popular since Arnold came on the scene in 1970s, women's bodybuilding reached its zenith in the early 1980s, when a handful of charismatic competitors such as Carla Dunlap, Rachel McLish, Gladys Portuguese, Mary Roberts, Laura Creavalle, and Cory Everson hit the scene. Not only were these woman strong and full of well-defined muscles (also known as being "ripped"), they were gorgeous—a marketing fact that made the mainstream press more eager to feature them on their pages.

Flex Facts

At 6 feet, 2 inches, 204 pounds, Nicole Bass, a popular Ms. Olympia competitor, is one of the largest female competitors ever officially weighed for a show. By contrast, Carla Dunlap—a far more accomplished bodybuilder—measured 5 feet, 3 inches, 126 pounds, proving that shape and symmetry are more important than size alone.

During the 1980s, female bodybuilding (particularly American female bodybuilding) emphasized a muscular yet *feminine* aesthetic—broad shoulders and back, narrow waist and hips. That all changed when the Americans and Europeans began competing against each other on a more regular basis. The Europeans tended to be bigger and more muscular—much more muscular!—and before you could say *latissimus dorsi*, the face of female bodybuilding had changed.

Since that change, female bodybuilding has lost much of its appeal and popularity. Said simply: many of the top professional female bodybuilders look like hyperdeveloped men in bikinis. More common now are what's called "fitness shows." Women who compete in said shows are muscular but not grotesque. However, these shows are more like watching a Miss America pageant because competitors wear high heels with their competition suits and perform routines heavy on dancing and gymnastics rather than on posing.

Weight a Minute

One of the reasons bodybuilding is so intimidating to aspiring competitors is the cartoonlike proportions of some of the high-profile names in the sport. It's something people don't like to talk about, but many bodybuilders' physiques have been affected by the abuse of anabolic steroids and/or plastic surgery. For those whose aspirations are a little different than the pros', *natural* bodybuilding contests are available. Drug testing is far stricter in such competitions.

Deidre's World

Powerlifting, a sport that became popular in the 1970s, was for a long time the ugly stepchild of bodybuilding. Oftentimes, powerlifting events were held late in the evening only after body-building competitions were over.

Early in Deidre's weight-lifting career, she seriously considered competing as a bodybuilder. However, as she learned more about the two sports, she decided powerlifting was the more pure sport because, unlike bodybuilding, it was not subjective. The goal in powerlifting is quite simple: the one who lifts the most wins.

Just as bodybuilding is a display of muscularity, powerlifting is a demonstration of strength. The disciplines in a powerlifting meet are three exercises we showed you already—the squat, bench press, and deadlift. A powerlifting competition consists of nine rounds of lifting per competitor—three attempts at each event. Because the highest successful lifts are added together, the winner is the one who totals the most weight.

If you're a 122-pound woman interested in competing at the world-class levels, here's what you're up against: when Deidre won her first world championship in 1995, her totals were squat, 303 pounds; bench press, 159 pounds; and deadlift, 336 pounds. By her peak, those numbers were up to 336, 187, and 370 pounds. If your aspirations are more along the line of local meets, half that will do just fine.

How It's Done

All three of these lifts are familiar to you by now, but the technique used in competition is very different from what we've recommended you do for your training. Here are the main differences:

◆ **Whenever possible, lifts are made *explosively*.** Momentum can make the difference between a successful lift and a miss.

◆ **You hold your breath.** The increased pressure caused by a valsalva maneuver (holding your breath while lifting) makes the lift easier. Unless you have learned this from a good coach, don't try this at home, because there is a tremendous increase in blood pressure generated when you hold your breath.

◆ **You squat below parallel.** When we described the squat in Chapter 7, we advocated bending your knees until they're parallel to the floor. Stop there in a powerlifting meet, and the lift is considered a no-go.

◆ **You arch your back while bench pressing.** In Chapter 9, we told you to always keep your back pressed into the bench when lifting to protect your lower back. Powerlifters arch their backs as much as possible to bring their chest up higher and shorten the range of motion of the lift. Again, their sole aim is to hoist as much weight as possible.

The mistake most lifters make in competitions is selecting a weight they can't manage on their opening attempt. This is potentially disastrous, because if you miss your opener, you can't change the weight. The rules dictate that you must stay with that same weight for your next two attempts. If you miss all three, it's all over. Deidre's openers were always a weight that she could do for two repetitions in the gym.

What's Done and Equipment You Need

There are two types of powerlifting events: those with equipment and those without. The equipment involved in powerlifting is nearly as restrictive as medieval armor. Once a lifter actually manages to wriggle into it, the lifting is the easy part. For the equipment-aided event, you'll need …

◆ **A squat suit.** This is a tight, stiff outfit made to give the lifter support during the squat. A good suit makes the squatting difficult, but it shoots you back to a standing position with comparative ease.

◆ **A belt.** Some belts offer the barest of support; others are so big they look like they could hoist a train wreck. Deidre first wore a belt called a lever belt that was fortified with hooks and a latch that looked like a harness for an ox. This sucker was so tight she could barely bend to get underneath the bar to squat.

◆ **Knee wraps.** These wraps are made of semi-elastic material that grudgingly gives an inch when you bend your knees. Along with the squat suit, the wraps are what give the lifter bounce when coming out of the squat. If you're eager to walk like a mummy, powerlifting knee wraps are for you.

◆ **Squat shoes.** These hard-soled shoes give the lifter support while squatting. The stiffness of the shoe restricts forward and backward sway as the lifter sets up with the weight on his or her back. The less sway, the more balance and control the lifter has.

◆ **A bench press shirt.** Made of either the same material as the squat suit or denim, these shirts are so tight it's virtually impossible to hold your arms at your side. Claustrophobics need not apply. An old powerlifting joke is that a good bench shirt can lift 40 or 50 pounds if you just lay it on the bench.

◆ **A unitard.** This is a one-piece wrestling singlet worn on top of the bench press shirt.

◆ **Wrist wraps.** Made from the same semi-elastic material as the knee wraps, these provide support during the bench press.

◆ **A deadlift suit.** Similar to a squat suit, the deadlift suit differs in that it's usually looser in the hips (so you can get down to the starting position).

◆ **Deadlift shoes.** These are flat, soft-soled shoes that bring the lifter closer to the

ground to decrease the distance the bar travels from the floor to the lifter's mid-thigh. Wrestling shoes or even ballet slippers are often used as well. (You haven't lived until you've seen a 275-pound bruiser wearing ballet slippers.)

Flex Facts

Those of you who paid attention in high school physics class will recognize that *powerlifting* is a misnomer. By definition, power is the rate at which work is done—the faster the movement, the greater the power. In the sport of powerlifting, all that matters is how much weight you lift—not how fast you lift it.

If you ever want to get the normally animated Deidre really hot and bothered, ask her about the joys of donning a squat suit. This torturous garment took two people 20 minutes to pull on and off. She's likely to wax poetic about the cuts in her legs where the suit dug in so tightly. (This is the hallmark of a good suit. If it slides up the legs, it decreases the amount of support through the quads and hips.) And she's sure to mention how the squat suit fit so well that her legs went numb. If any of this sounds like fun, you're probably ready to launch your career as a powerlifter.

Of course, if powerlifting intrigues you but the equipment doesn't, you could be a candidate for a *raw* meet, where the only equipment required is a unitard and the only other paraphernalia allowed is a standard weight-lifting belt. The good thing about raw meets is that lifters tend to be far more careful in their selection of weight attempts. Wearing a squat suit or a bench press shirt often gives lifters a false sense of security, and they often choose weights beyond their capabilities. This, of course, is a great way to get injured.

Let's look at the three disciplines a bit more carefully.

The Squat

The squat is the first event in a powerlifting meet—and the most nerve-racking, primarily because you wear the most equipment and feel the most vulnerable standing under all that weight. It is also the lift that requires the lifter to be almost perfect in terms of form and technique—especially when the weight approaches double or triple body weight. As we mentioned, for the squat attempt to be deemed good, you must lower your body until your hip joint is below your knee joint.

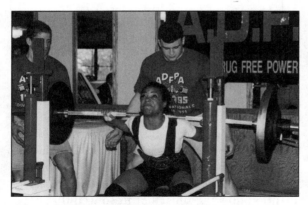

Deidre squatting in competition—start.

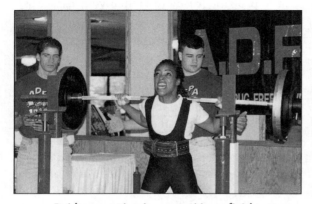

Deidre squatting in competition—finish.

Here are the elements required for a near-perfect squat during a competition:

◆ **The setup.** How the lifter approaches and gets underneath the bar is probably the most psychological aspect of the lift. Approach with fear, and more often than not you're likely to miss. Approach with a mixture of nervousness and confidence, and you'll nail it almost every time.

◆ **The walk out.** After you've come under the bar, you must stand with the weight on your back and walk backward so you don't hit the squat racks. The best way to walk out is to use the least number of steps possible. The more steps you take, the more the weight bounces on your back, throwing off your balance and rhythm. It also gives you too much time to think about just how much weight you're carrying on your back. The best walkout is to take one step back and stop.

◆ **The squat.** When you've stopped moving your feet and are focused and steady, you are given the signal to squat. The best way to begin the descent is to hear the signal, take a deep breath, and squat. Some people take several quick, shallow breaths before squatting, which just wastes time and energy. One breath and squat is all you need. Basically, the more time you have the weight on your back, the heavier it begins to feel.

The Bench

The bench press is the second event and, like the squat, requires a substantial bit of technical precision. Here are the basics:

◆ The lifter brings her feet as far back toward her head as possible to arch her back.

◆ A spotter lifts the bar off the rack and hands it to the lifter.

- The lifter takes a deep breath and lowers the bar until it touches her chest. Only after it comes to a complete stop can the grunting competitor press the weight off her chest. Any bouncing of the bar or uneven extension of the arms, and the lift is disallowed.

The Deadlift

There's an old powerlifting adage that says, "The meet doesn't start till the bar hits the floor." This sage piece of lifting wisdom means meets are often won and lost with the deadlift—the final lift of the day.

Deidre won many meets where she trailed after the squat and bench press, only to pull it out at the end. In fact, her lifting partner and friend, four-time national champion Jacqueline Davis, once won a national meet by outlifting her competitor by 75 pounds in the deadlift!

Here's what to expect during the deadlift:

- First your hands will be covered in chalk to help you grip the bar. Your shins and thighs will be similarly covered in baby powder to help the bar slide up your legs more easily. (Mix up the two, and expect the bar to slip out of your hands or stick to your thighs.)
- Grip the bar as described in Chapter 8 or in a variation known as the *sumo* position.
- Take a deep breath, and pull like an ox plowing a hard field. The lifter is required to stand fully erect before receiving the "down" call from the head official.

Bar Talk

The **sumo** deadlift, which Deidre used in competition, is when the lifter takes a wide stance and places her hands inside her legs.

So there you have it: familiar lifts done with unfamiliar technique. With all their hooting and hollering, chalk-smattered and often bulky bodies, powerlifting meets can be an intimidating place. (Although the raw meets are generally a bit more laid-back, we hesitate to call them civilized.) In either case, many meets have a novice division, which is a great way to check out this little-known sport.

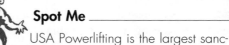

Spot Me

USA Powerlifting is the largest sanctioning organization in the sport, though many others exist. *Powerlifting USA* magazine is the bible of powerlifting and a good resource for information on upcoming meets and coverage of the sport.

The Big Boys

The sport of Olympic weight lifting, sometimes known simply as weight lifting, is better known to the general public than powerlifting due to the exposure it receives every 4 years during the Olympics. The fact that very few Americans distinguish themselves on the international level tends to keep it in the athletic closet. (The Eastern Europeans dominate the sport.) Compared to powerlifting, there's a minimum of equipment—only a belt, knee wraps, and wrist wraps. The competitor wears a singlet and hard-soled shoes.

The two lifts used in competition are known as the snatch and the clean and jerk. Each competitor is allowed three attempts in each lift. The sum of the lifter's best snatches and best clean and jerks is the lifter's total.

The reason we've not described these lifts in previous chapters is because there's little justification for anyone but a competitive lifter to do them. If you're inspired to try to learn these lifts, a knowledgeable coach is a must. These lifts are performed explosively, and because they require you to hoist the weight over your head, there's a substantial risk of injury. In fact, one of the exciting aspects of this sport—other than the incredible totals these lifters put up—is the explosive speed and power a lifter must possess to be able to leap under the weight. Even the superheavyweights, men who resemble rhinos more than athletes, possess a startling grace once they grasp these seemingly immovable pounds of iron.

To find out more, surf over to USA Weightlifting through their website at www.usaweightlifting.org. They list everything from equipment to meets to coaches for the sport. To find out more about the snatch and clean and jerk lifts, read on.

The Snatch

The more technical and more explosive of the two lifts, the snatch looks like a great way to dislocate both of your shoulders. Done correctly, it's a picture-book demonstration of grace, speed, and power.

The snatch is performed in one continuous movement. The bar is brought from the platform to a position overhead using one fluid motion. The lifter pulls the bar up from the platform. When the bar reaches the lifter's chest, he or she then leaps into a squat position under the bar, securing it overhead with arms held straight. Once the lifter has accomplished that impracticable move, he or she must stand upright. Sounds impossible? It almost is.

The Clean and Jerk

Although this lift sounds like one of those goofy Jim Carrey movies, in fact this is a deadly serious lift in which competitors hoist far more weight than the snatch.

As the name implies, the clean and jerk is a two-part movement. For the clean, the lifter must yank the weight from the platform to the shoulders in one motion and then stand erect. The jerk part is where the lifter thrusts the bar from his shoulders to a position overhead in one motion while splitting his legs. If he's made it that far, the lifter must put his wobbly legs together and stand motionless. After he gets the okay sign, it's time to send the weight crashing back to Earth where it belongs.

The Least You Need to Know

◆ If you love to lift as well as compete, you should check out one (or all) of the three competitive avenues: bodybuilding, powerlifting, or Olympic-style weight lifting.

◆ Bodybuilding requires countless hours in the gym to build a muscular, symmetrical, and lean body.

◆ Powerlifting involves three common exercises, but with uncommonly heavy weight.

◆ Olympic weight lifting uses two technically challenging lifts in competition.

In This Chapter

- ◆ Lifting will improve your game
- ◆ Preventing injury is as important as anything else
- ◆ Exercising for your sport

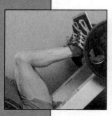
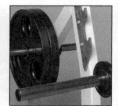
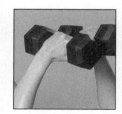
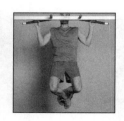
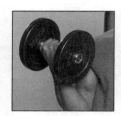
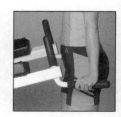

Chapter 18

Lift Well, Play Hard

Whether you're a jockey, synchronized swimmer, or badminton player, virtually every athlete can benefit from increased strength. In this chapter, we help you design strength-training routines aimed at helping your performance in a variety of sports, from golf to football. What may surprise you are the similarities in how we train athletes for such diverse sports. Obviously, the demands of these sports are very different, and the muscles that need to be trained vary from sport to sport, but surprisingly, the techniques used in the weight room will not.

Specificity of training, the concept that exercises should be based on the physiological demands encountered during the performance of a sport, is one of the most misunderstood items in exercise science. Some strength coaches advocate using sports-specific exercises in the weight room that mimic the movement used in your sport. The theory seems sound: by copying such movements, you help develop strength in that particular movement. While that seems like a logical line of reasoning, many experts think it may, in fact, be counterproductive.

Another buzzword that has gained considerable popularity over the past few years is *functional* training, in which the lifter performs exercises in an intentionally unstable position such as on one leg or precariously balanced on a wobble board or stability ball. Because it's challenging and different, such training has become all the rage, but we question its validity for most athletes (or nonathletes). Remember—just because something's hard, and just because it gets easier as you practice it—doesn't mean it's beneficial. The theory behind this type of training is that it increases your "core" strength while strengthening your muscles in movement patterns that can't be duplicated on a machine or with conventional weight-training exercises. Again, we question the physiological basis for this method. As we explained earlier, muscles only respond if they're overloaded. If you're not on a stable base, you can't recruit as many muscle fibers and, therefore, can't gain as much strength. True—it is important for an athlete to work on core strength and balance—just not while they're trying to get stronger. Get strong and then practice your sports-specific skills and movements.

Can You Be More Specific?

Specificity is much like pregnancy—it either is or it isn't. For example, specific training for a basketball player could be practicing his jump shot, not shooting a weighted medicine ball. In fact, by attempting to mimic a precise sports movement such as swinging a baseball bat or golf club, you can undo countless hours of skill training. You see, the neuromuscular pathways that allow your brain to tell your muscles exactly what to do—and how to do it—take countless hours of practice. In turn, the use of added resistance (for example, the medicine ball) when copying such movements can disturb that motor memory.

> **Bar Talk**
>
> **Specificity of training** is a well-accepted physiological theory that suggests that adaptations made during training depend on the type of training used. For instance, if you want to become a faster runner, the most appropriate way to accomplish this is by running, not by walking in the park or riding a bike.

Princeton University's Matt Brzycki, author of *A Practical Approach to Strength Training* (McGraw Hill, 1998), is one of the most outspoken strength critics of copying sports movements in the weight room. Says Mr. Brzycki, "Strength training should not be done in a manner that mimics or apes a particular movement pattern. A stronger muscle can produce more force; if you can produce more force, you'll require less effort and be able to perform the

skill more quickly, more accurately, and more efficiently. But again, that is provided that you've practiced enough in a correct manner so that you'll be more skillful in applying that force."

Just as we don't advocate different training techniques in the weight room for men and women or the young and the old, there's no reason to train athletes from different sports using different techniques. Good weight room form for a cyclist is good weight room form for a tennis player. What should, and will, vary is the selection of exercises because the muscles used differ from sport to sport. That's where we *customize* the programs. For example, a kayaker will do more upper body work than a runner, but the upper body work they perform they'll do exactly the same.

A few years ago, Jonathan attended a seminar held by John Philbin, an assistant strength and conditioning coach with the NFL's Washington Redskins. What surprised many in attendance was that although the Redskins vary their exercises from position to position (no sense in worrying about the throwing arm of the free safety), the form used is exactly the same for any and all of the athletes. Typically, a lithe cornerback can bench press far less than a burly linebacker, but the exercise is executed exactly the same way.

Improved performance is an obvious reason for an athlete—weekend warrior or professional—to hit the weight room, but it may not be the most important one. In fact, injury prevention is probably the biggest benefit from a solid off-season training regimen. After all, it doesn't matter how talented you are if you're on the sidelines nursing an injury. Barry Chait, former assistant strength and conditioning coach with the NFL's New York Jets, stresses that, "Though we obviously try everything possible to make the players bigger, faster, and stronger, our primary goal is to ensure they make it through the game in one piece. That means never taking any chances in the weight room, and it means working on less glamorous muscles like those in the neck."

Years ago, many athletes used to resist weight lifting for fear of becoming muscle-bound. (One can only imagine how many more homers Mickey Mantle would have hit had he touched a weight during his career. Even if he didn't hit any more dingers, he would have hit them much farther, and he may have avoided the debilitating leg injuries that curtailed his career.) Now that the muscle-bound myth has gone the way of the eight-track tape, many athletes still shy away from the weight room, fearing that they'll lose valuable training time they could better spend practicing their sport.

Certainly we agree that all the strength in the world can't make up for the lack of a sport-specific skill; however, there's no reason to choose between the two. By now, we hope we've convinced you that a sensible lifting program doesn't need to take more than 30 to 45 minutes per gym visit.

Because very few athletes compete year-round—Steffi Graf, where have you gone?—there's no reason to have the same program in season as you do out of season.

Here's how it works: in the off season, your primary goal is to get as strong as possible. During the season, however, you should aim to maintain your strength. If you try to keep up the same schedule while you compete as you did in the off season, you're begging for over-training injuries. Of course, if you lay off your lifting completely, you'll quickly undo all the good you've done. Aim for two or three lifting sessions per week in the off season and once a week for maintenance in season. Try to keep your in-season workout on a different day than a hard sports workout and at least a few days away from a race.

Stick Out Your Neck

Strong neck muscles (primarily the sternocleidomastoid, scalenes, splenius capitus, and splenius cervicis) may not be of any particular use to a golfer, but they can be invaluable for anyone whose sport has a risk of head and neck injuries such as football players or wrestlers. Even a cyclist will benefit from added neck strength. (If you don't believe us, check out Jonathan's collection of cracked helmets from bicycle crashes he's been in.) On the other hand, a golfer or kayaker would be wise to focus on grip strength far more than a swimmer or runner.

Weight a Minute

Although neck muscles aren't very glamorous, they're important for athletes in contact sports or those who are in danger of head injuries. In other words, if you wear a helmet for your sport, you'll probably decrease your risk of injury by doing a few simple neck exercises.

Some gyms have specially designed neck machines, and others have a harness you can wear on your head to do various exercises. We've described the simplest way of doing them, which is with manual resistance—you press against your head with your hand. Not very high-tech, but reliable and effective.

Here is how to properly perform neck flexion:

1. Sit in a chair with back support.
2. While looking forward, place the palm of your dominant hand on your forehead.

3. Bend your head forward, chin toward your chest. Resist the movement of your head by applying backward pressure to your forehead with your hand.
4. Slowly return to the starting position.

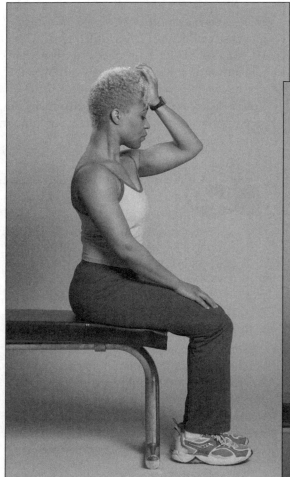

Neck flexion start/finish position.

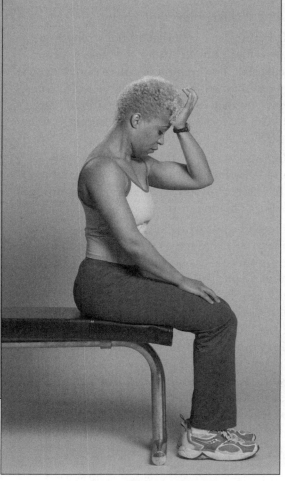

Neck flexion middle position.

Here is how to properly perform neck extension:

1. Sit in a chair with back support.
2. While looking forward, place the palm of your dominant hand on the back of your head.

3. Bend your head backward so you're looking up toward the ceiling. As you do so, resist the movement by applying forward pressure to the back of your head with your hand.
4. Slowly return to the starting position.

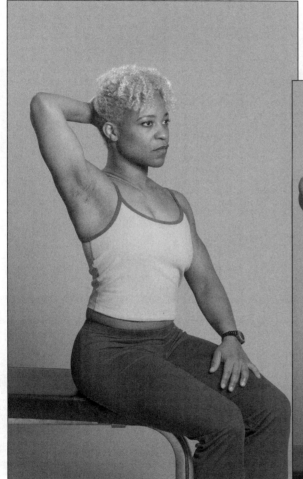

Neck extension start/finish position.

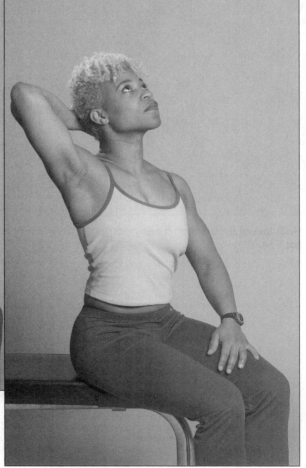

Neck extension middle position.

Here is how to properly perform a neck lateral flexion:

1. Sit in a chair with back support.
2. While looking forward, place the palm of your hand on the side of your head.

3. Bend your head sideways, being sure to keep your nose facing straight (not toward the ceiling). As you do so, resist the movement by applying pressure to the side of your head in the opposite direction.
4. Slowly return to the starting position. Repeat on the other side.

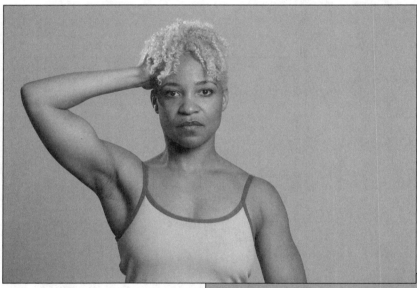

Neck lateral flexion start/finish position.

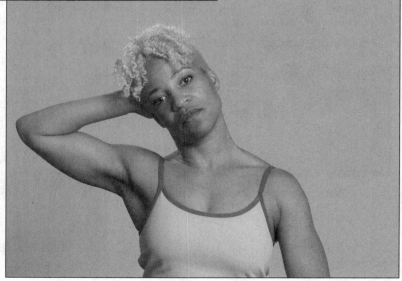

Neck lateral flexion middle position.

What follows is a list of exercises based on the demands of a particular sport. Remember that our selection of the exercises is specific to the sport, but the form used is the same regardless of the sport.

Running

Running more than a half-mile or so is primarily an aerobic activity, but even long-distance runners can benefit from improved muscular strength. The added strength helps you power up hills, but the main reason for runners to lift is injury prevention. For example …

◆ Patellar tendinitis, an inflammation of the connective tissue around the kneecap, is a common running injury that can be prevented or minimized with improved quadriceps strength.

◆ Hamstring strains, which are as common to veteran runners as Gatorade at road races, can be prevented with a sound strength-training program as well.

◆ Trochanteric bursitis is another condition common in runners, cross-country skiers, and ballet dancers that can be kept at bay with weight training. When the *bursa* becomes inflamed, the result is a deep, burning pain on the *trochanter* itself or, less often, down the side of the thigh. Treatment of this condition—aside from rest, ice, stretching, and anti-inflammatories—involves strengthening all the gluteal muscles.

Bar Talk

A **bursa** is a sac found between muscle and bone or bone and tendon that helps decrease friction. The **trochanter** is the prominent bone found on either side of the hip.

Another concern of distance runners that can be improved with a sound weight program is the imbalance between the hamstrings and the quadriceps. Most distance runners have well-developed hamstrings but weak quadriceps. Strengthening the quads can help prevent running injuries and helps restore the proper balance.

Finally, while running is obviously primarily a lower body activity, you'd be surprised at how much your upper body contributes. If you don't believe us, try running up a hill with your hands behind your back. Large muscles are a hindrance; strong muscles help you run faster.

The following table lists specific body parts and exercises that are good to perform together if you are a runner.

Body Part	Exercises
Legs and hips	Squat or leg press
	Leg curl
	Abduction
	Adduction
	Standing calf raise
	Seated calf raise
Back	Pull-ups (assisted, if necessary)
Chest	Dips (assisted, if necessary)
Shoulders	Shoulder press
Arms	Seated biceps curl
	Triceps pushdown
Midsection	Reverse crunches
	Crunches
	Oblique crunches
	Back raises

Cycling

Many of the injuries among cyclists are a result of improper mechanics rather than muscular weakness. Some of these injuries include patellar tendinitis, quadriceps tendinitis, pes anserinus bursitis, chondromalacia patella, and iliotibial band syndrome.

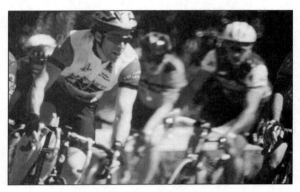

Jonathan hard at work.

Just as with runners, cyclists often suffer from muscular imbalances, though their imbalance is the opposite of what runners encounter. Jonathan's quads have served him well through hundreds of bicycle races (as well as a few races up the stairs of the Empire State Building), but by comparison, his hamstrings are woefully weak. A good dose of leg curls could help remedy his problem. (We hope he'll read this chapter and act accordingly.)

As in the case of runners, added extra body bulk can be detrimental, but upper body strength is necessary when sprinting and riding out of the saddle while you're powering your way up a steep hill. In addition, midsection strength can help give you a good, solid base for all those miles in the saddle. Back exercises can help reverse the hunched posture caused by all those hours of riding. Finally, don't forget those neck exercises we mentioned earlier.

The following table is a sample program for the cycling fans.

Body Part	Exercises
Legs and hips	Squat or leg press
	Leg extension
	Leg curl
	Standing calf raise
	Seated calf raise
Back	Pull-ups (assisted, if necessary)
	Upright row
Chest	Dips
Shoulders	Military press
Arms	Seated biceps curl
	Triceps pushdown
Midsection	Reverse crunches
	Crunches
	Oblique crunches
	Back raises
Neck	Extension
	Flexion
	Lateral flexion

Tennis

If you have any questions whether strength can help a tennis player, you need look no further than the Amazonlike Williams sisters, Venus and Serena. These tall, powerfully built young women regularly serve at speeds comparable to men on the pro tour. Equally as impressive is their all-court athleticism. This combination of speed and power has propelled them to the top of their sport.

Tennis and other racquet sports require good upper body strength for hitting the ball; abdominal and oblique strength for twisting of the torso; and leg strength to help get you to the ball. When Andre Agassi rededicated himself to tennis en route to winning the 1999 French Open, he credited his rigorous weight program for giving him that extra *oomph* on the ball.

The most common injuries associated with tennis are lateral epicondylitis (known as tennis elbow) and to a much lesser extent, medial epicondylitis (known as golfer's elbow but also seen in tennis players). The best way to prevent and/or resolve these injuries is to strengthen the muscles of the forearm with wrist flexion and extension exercises.

The following exercises should keep you on the court and hitting hard. You still might not be able to give either of the Williams sisters much to worry about, but you'll certainly look impressive on the way to and from the court.

Body Part	Exercises
Legs and hips	Lunges
	Abduction
	Adduction
	Standing calf raise
Back	Bent row
	Lat pull-down
Chest	Pec deck
	Bench press
Shoulders	Lateral raise
	Military press
	Internal rotation
	External rotation
Arms	Seated biceps curl
	Triceps kickback
	Wrist curls

Body Part	Exercises
Midsection	Reverse crunch
	Crunch
	Rotary torso
	Back raise

Golf

Okay, so you don't need to be the world's greatest athlete to excel in golf, and you're not likely to see the paunchy Phil Mickelson on the cover of *Ironman* magazine any time soon. On the other hand, we've already told you increased strength increases club-head speed and drive distance, so golfers certainly can benefit from a strength-training program. And one has to look no further than the game's greatest player today, Tiger Woods, who has lifted weights for years. Is there any correlation between his mammoth drives and his strength? We certainly think there is.

Muscles of particular importance to golfers include the gripping muscles of the hands and forearms, the obliques for twisting during the shot, and the muscles of the arms and shoulders to help power the ball. In the routine that follows, we pay particular attention to these body parts as well as a thorough midsection routine to power your torso through your stroke.

As for injuries, medial epicondylitis is much more common in golfers than it is in tennis players. Again, the best way to prevent and/or resolve it is by strengthening the forearm muscles with wrist flexion and extension exercises. In addition, back pain among golfers is common due to the fast, twisting motion. Strengthening your abs, obliques, and lower back can keep you on course. (Bad pun, but it's true.)

Here's a solid lifting program for golfers. By the way, ditch the cart and walk instead—you'll up your fitness quotient considerably.

Body Part	Exercises
Legs and hips	Leg press
	Leg curl
Back	Lat pull-down
Chest	Bench press
Shoulders	Lateral raise
	Military press
Arms	Seated biceps curl
	Triceps pushdown
	Wrist curls
Midsection	Reverse crunches
	Crunches
	Rotary torso
	Back raise

Baseball

John Kruk, the portly former all-star first base-man for the Philadelphia Phillies, once said, "I'm not an athlete, I'm a baseball player." Certainly he wasn't the first player to prove you don't need be a stud athlete to make it on the diamond. Fast-forward to the twenty-first century, and it has been clearly demonstrated that being a well-rounded athlete can only enhance your game if you have the requisite skills and hand-eye coordination.

Power aside, baseball is a game of spurts and starts with a healthy dose of arm strain thrown in. Arm injuries such as rotator cuff tendinitis and shoulder dislocations can be prevented or improved with a proper strengthening program. Midsection strength can help avoid back injuries from the repetitive motion of swinging a bat. And both upper and lower body strength can improve one's arm and bat speed. Remember that if the bat moves faster, the ball goes farther.

The following exercises should keep you on the field. And if you "got no game," they'll at least have you looking more athletic than the hard-hitting yet portly Mr. Kruk.

Body Part	Exercises
Legs and hips	Squat or leg press
	Leg curl
	Abduction
	Adduction
Back	Pull-ups (assisted, if necessary)
	Bent row
Chest	Bench press
Shoulders	Military press
	Internal rotation
	External rotation
Arms	Seated biceps curl
	Triceps pushdown
	Wrist curls
Midsection	Reverse crunches
	Crunches
	Rotary torso
	Back raise

Basketball

Ever know a guy who could shoot the lights out during warm-ups or win any game of H-O-R-S-E but could barely score a point during the game? How about the player who excels early in the game, but whose jump shot always hits the front of the rim as the game goes on? Sure, you need to be able to shoot the ball, but if you don't have the physical ability to run up and down the court and establish your position in the paint, all the skill in the world won't do you any good.

Watch an NBA basketball game, and you can't help but marvel at the incredible athleticism exhibited on the court. Speed, strength, and flexibility are all necessary physical attributes of a successful player. You may not be playing in the pros any time soon, but to excel at the weekend pickup game at the Y requires those same physical abilities.

Strong legs are essential to establishing position in the low post and jumping. Upper body strength can help your jumping as well and is necessary when shooting and boxing out for a rebound.

In the injury-prevention realm, anterior cruciate ligament tears are an all-too-common injury among basketball players (especially women, in part due to the width of their hips). Once again, increased quadriceps strength can help prevent or minimize such injuries.

These exercises should help fortify you on and off the court.

Body Part	Exercises
Legs and hips	Squat or leg press
	Leg extension
	Leg curl
	Standing calf raise
	Seated calf raise
Back	Lat pull-down
Chest	Bench press
Shoulders	Military press
Arms	Seated biceps curl
	Triceps pushdown
Midsection	Reverse crunches
	Crunches
	Oblique crunches
	Back raise

Swimming

Swimming fast requires a tremendous amount of skill and strength. The chiseled physique and V-shaped taper of an elite swimmer should leave little doubt about that. The muscles used vary from stroke to stroke, but it's safe to say swimmers need good chest, shoulder, and back strength as well as abdominal strength for stability when rotating to breathe. Leg strength for the kick is also essential.

Swimmers, especially elite swimmers, are extremely flexible, which affords them enormous range of motion (ROM) while they propel themselves through the water. This flexibility, coupled with overdevelopment of the muscles of the front of their upper body (pecs and anterior delts), puts swimmers at risk for rotator cuff injuries, tendinitis, muscle tears, and shoulder dislocations. A weight-training routine that emphasizes strengthening the upper back muscles and the posterior deltoid muscles decreases the muscle imbalance often associated with these aquatic types. Strengthening the rotator cuff muscles decreases the risk of the shoulder injuries so common to hard-core swimmers.

The thing that all athletes should keep in mind—especially those whose sport depends on a greater-than-average range of motion—is that strength training does not inhibit flexibility as long as you lift through a full range of motion. Strength training decreases that risk without decreasing your flexibility.

Here's a regimen that should make Summer Sanders proud.

Body Part	Exercises
Legs and hips	Leg press
	Leg curl
Back	Lat pull-down
	Upright row

continues

continued

Body Part	Exercises
Chest	Bench press
Shoulders	Military press
	Lateral raise
	Reverse flye
	Front raise
	Internal rotation
	External rotation
Arms	Seated biceps curl
	Triceps kickback
Midsection	Reverse crunch
	Crunch
	Rotary torso
	Back raise

Skiing and Snowboarding

A successful downhill or slalom skier needs strong quads and glutes to hold the tucked position. In addition, upper-body strength is helpful when you're working your poles through bumpy terrain.

Just as with cyclists, there are two types of skiers: those who have crashed and those who haven't crashed *yet*. For that reason alone, the greater stability stronger muscles give you can help minimize injuries in the event of a crash. Quadriceps strength is also important in the prevention of knee injuries that can be brought on by the twisting and pivoting motion of hammering downhill.

Here's a list of exercises that will get you ready.

Body Part	Exercises
Legs and hips	Squat or leg press
	Lunges
	Leg curl
	Leg extension
	Abduction
	Adduction
Back	Lat pull-down
Chest	Bench press
Shoulders	Military press
Arms	Seated biceps curl
	Triceps pushdown
Midsection	Reverse crunch
	Crunch
	Oblique crunch
	Back raise

Skating

Both ice skating and its newfangled dry-land cousin, in-line skating, require quite a bit of leg strength, as well as more upper-body and midsection strength than you might realize.

Obviously, the muscles of your legs are the engine that propels you forward; however, strength in your lower back and abs enables you to stay in a tight tuck as you work your arms to help keep you rolling along. Several elite bicycle racers have made the transition from cycling to speed skating because of the similarities between the physical demands of the two sports.

Another thing cyclists and skaters have in common is that they both inevitably hit the ground sooner or later. That's our way of reminding you not to skip the wrist and neck exercises we recommend.

Here's a program catered to keeping you swift, fit, and healthy.

Body Part	Exercises
Legs and hips	Squat or leg press
	Lunge
	Abduction
	Adduction
Back	Lat pull-down
Chest	Bench press
Shoulders	Military press
Arms	Seated biceps curl
	Triceps pushdown
	Wrist curls
Midsection	Reverse crunch
	Crunch
	Oblique crunch
	Back raise
Neck	Flexion
	Extension
	Lateral flexion

Kayaking

Line up the competition at a kayak race, and you're bound to see lots of broad, muscular, V-shaped torsos atop spindly legs. Paddlers spend hours at a time working away with their backs, shoulders, and arms while their legs remain safely tucked away. (Your legs actually are instrumental in a sound stroke, but they act mostly as stabilizers instead of sources of speed.)

There's no need for a paddler to spend a lot of time on his or her legs, as you'll see from the program we've designed. On the other hand, hours of twisting the torso are facilitated by strong obliques, abs, and lower back muscles. The muscles of the back and shoulders provide most of the power in the stroke, so that's where we place our primary emphasis.

The most common injuries among paddlers involve the rotator cuff, so don't forget those internal and external rotation exercises.

The following exercises may not float your boat, but they'll definitely get it moving through the water faster.

Body Part	Exercises
Legs and hips	Leg extension
	Leg curl
Back	Pull-ups (assisted, if necessary)
	Dumbbell rows
Chest	Bench press
	Dips (assisted, if necessary)
Shoulders	Military press
	Lateral raise
	Internal rotation
	External rotation
Arms	Seated biceps curl
	Triceps pushdown
Midsection	Reverse crunch
	Crunch
	Oblique crunch
	Back raise

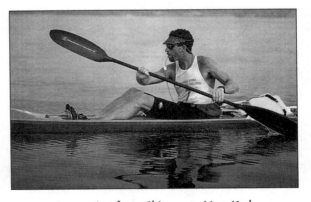

Joe, racing from Chicago to New York.

Martial Arts and Boxing

Mention training for boxing to most people, and they'll probably think of a regimen of countless sit-ups and hard roadwork, as well as punching slabs of beef. All those are fine, but we prefer you pound blocks of tofu, because overgrazing is a big problem in our country.

Martial arts? With more and more people getting involved in Asian arts such as boxing and kickboxing, there's still room for some more-conventional training methods. Whether it's the real thing or classes, strengthening your body can help you perform better.

While we are all in favor of you waxing hundreds of cars a week (see *The Karate Kid*) or meditating under frigid waterfalls, our workout regimen has you building strong legs (for fancy footwork), strong shoulders (for packing a punch), and a strong midsection and neck (in case you're on the receiving end of one of those blows).

Here's a workout strategy that should keep you in fighting shape.

Body Part	Exercises
Legs and hips	Squat or leg press
	Leg curl
	Abduction
	Adduction
Back	Pull-ups (assisted, if necessary)
	Dumbbell rows
Chest	Bench press
	Dips (assisted, if necessary)
Shoulders	Military press
	Lateral raise
Arms	Seated biceps curl
	Triceps kickback
Midsection	Reverse crunch
	Crunch
	Oblique crunch
	Back raise
Neck	Flexion
	Extension
	Lateral flexion

The Least You Need to Know

◆ No matter what the sport, improving your strength will help you on and off the court.

◆ All the talent in the world won't help if you're sidelined with an injury.

◆ Neck exercises may not sound exciting, but they're important for sports that involve crashes or contact.

In This Chapter

- ◆ Lifting, running, and being merry
- ◆ Calculating your pace
- ◆ Spinning, stepping, and dancing

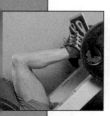 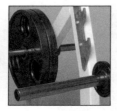 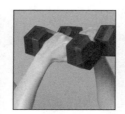 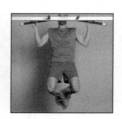 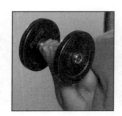 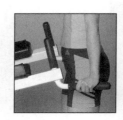

Chapter 19

Mix It Up

If you haven't guessed by now, we're kind of keen on weight training as a way to improve your health and fitness. While we've extolled the virtues of weight training for the better part of 18 chapters, we would be remiss if we didn't stress that aerobic exercise is a necessary complement to weight training. In other words, if you want to get strong, lift weights; if you want to be truly fit, add cardiovascular (CV) exercise into the mix.

It may come as a revelation to most of you, but it's a misconception that aerobic exercise tones and firms muscle. Aerobic exercise helps you decrease your level of body fat, which helps improve the muscle definition by thinning out the layer of fat that obscures the muscles. Weight training is what makes the muscles worth looking at. Theoretically, you can be thin from doing tons of aerobic exercises, yet still be flabby and/or weak. To achieve a balanced physique, you must include both aerobics and weight training in your routine.

Take Deidre's early foray into the world of endorphins. She started off doing aerobics without weight training; then she weight trained without aerobics. Next she did both, though she paid no attention to nutrition. Finally, she hit pay dirt when she combined aerobic exercise, weight training, and proper nutrition. Not only did she look strong, lean, and muscular, she felt great as well. (It was only after she'd been competing as a powerlifter for several years that her body said, "No more!")

Unlike weight lifting, there are an infinite number of aerobic activities that you can choose from: cross-country skiing, swimming, in-line skating, hiking, running, cycling (on- or off-road), stair climbing, and walking. Given this wide range of activities, almost anyone who enjoys working up a sweat can find something he or she derives joy from.

Spot Me _____
During the first 20 minutes of cardio-vascular activity, carbohydrates are the primary energy source. Aerobic activity that lasts longer than 20 minutes begins to metabolize fat for energy. While short, intense bursts of exercise can help your car-diovascular system, moderately paced (not slow), longer workouts are preferable if your goal is to burn fat.

This isn't to suggest you have to become a marathon man like Joe or Jonathan. Consider one of Deidre's friends who would rather have rusty tacks driven under her fingernails than exercise aerobically indoors. Instead of making it a dreaded chore, she cycles or blades from her apartment in Brooklyn to her office in Manhattan and back several times a week. Inte-grating her exercise into her workday leaves her feeling fit, virtuous, and on time. She's lucky enough to have access to a shower at her job, and she brings a stack of work clothes in every Monday.

Deidre, on the other hand, prefers doing her aerobic workouts indoors rather than dealing with traffic, unruly dogs, and/or the aggressive cyclists one often finds in Brooklyn's Prospect Park. Because she is basically a fast-twitch muscle person—no genetic predisposition to endurance in that muscular body—long periods of aerobic activity are not her idea of fun. In turn, unless she's jogging through a flowery meadow to soothe her urban soul, she'd just as soon escape to a treadmill in the gym and grind away as she listens to her Walkman.

Jonathan is another case study. He'll exercise wherever he can find pavement, a treadmill, or virtually any piece of aerobic exercise equip-ment. Tell him you have a new machine called a floppy-loop that works your anterior hip abductors, and he's sure to give it a try. He'll train in any kind of weather and at any time of the day or night. He loves it when it's 90 degrees; he loves it when it's raining. Call him noble, call him maladjusted, or just call him a true exercise junkie.

Joe is in the Jonathan camp. You'll find Joe wherever kayaks lurk. He also has a penchant for climbing mountains and/or running or biking on trails. By the way, did we mention snowshoe marathons and winter triathlons? In fact, pick a cardio exercise that is long, hard, or stupid, and Joe's generally game. (In fact, on Jonathan's insistence, he trained for and competed on the Concept II rowing machine in an indoor regatta known as The St. Valentine's Day Massacre.)

Before we continue, let's define what we mean by aerobic exercise for adequate cardio-vascular fitness and weight loss. This is any activity that sustains an elevated heart rate for at least 20 minutes, preferably at least 3 or 4 times per week. Once you're comfortably able to sustain 20 to 30 minutes of a CV activity, try to extend your aerobic exercise session to 45 minutes. Of course, don't try to do this all at once. Rather, up the ante 5 minutes per week. What we really hope to avoid is you attempt-ing more than you can handle at one time. That's one way people get frustrated and stop.

Lub Dub: Heart Rates

To get a good cardiovascular workout, it's help-ful to know how hard to push yourself. (Going too slow loses the training benefit; training too hard is often unnecessary, counterproductive, or even dangerous.) As a result, the best way to monitor your pace is by figuring out your heart rate and knowing at what level of exertion to train.

Although it initially may seem complicated, figuring out your heart rate while you exercise is quite easy. In fact, before you know it, you'll be monitoring your heart rate like Jonathan. A number-cruncher at heart, he often checks his heart rate after a shower, while watching a scary movie, or when waiting in line at the bank. (Please don't ask why he does this. While he's extremely knowledgeable on all aspects of fitness, he is rather, how shall we say, unique.)

To make the heart-rate-number-crunching game worth your while, you'll need to know a few basics:

◆ To maximize weight loss, you want to exercise at 60 to 75 percent of your maximal heart rate (MHR).

◆ For cardiovascular fitness, you want to increase this to about 85 percent of your MHR. Elite athletes, such as Olympic sprinters, often push the envelope and exercise at nearly 100 percent of their MHR.

Figure It Out

The simplest way to determine whether you're exercising aerobically or *anaerobically* is the talk test. If you can carry on a conversation with your training mate while you're jogging around the park, you're training aerobically; you may be huffing and puffing, but you can be understood and respond without gasping for breath. If your partner asks, "How ya doin'?" and you reply like a breathless mugger wearing a ski mask, well, you're in the anaerobic range.

Bar Talk

Literally speaking, **anaerobic** means "in the absence of oxygen." When the term *anaerobic* is used relating to exercise, it refers to exercises such as weight lifting that do not require oxygen. Weight lifting is considered an anaerobic activity.

You can also use what is called your rate of perceived exertion (RPE). This charted rate attempts to quantify for you how hard you're working when you're exercising. This is very often used with patients who are participating in cardiac rehabilitation after suffering a heart attack or cardiovascular surgery. The RPE scale is imperfect because it's so subjective, but it can be a useful tool to go along with monitoring your heart rate.

The following is the scale for rate of perceived exertion (RPE):

0	Nothing at all
0.5	Very, very weak
1	Very weak
2	Weak
3	Moderate
4	Somewhat strong
5	Strong
6	Strong
7	Very strong
8	Very strong
9	Very strong
10	Very, very strong
•	Maximal

If you don't have anyone by your side to talk to and fear being considered a nut job carrying on a one-sided conversation, you can use two formulas to figure out what your target heart rate should be during your workout.

The first formula to figure out your THR is as follows:

1. Subtract your age from 220 to find your predicted maximum heart rate (MHR).
2. Multiply your MHR by 60 percent. This represents the low end of your target heart rate.
3. Multiply your MHR by 85 percent. This is the high end of your target heart rate.

The second, more-accurate way to figure your *target heart rate* during aerobic activity is called the Karvonen formula. First, you need to record your resting heart rate (RHR). To get an accurate reading, take your pulse first thing in the morning before you get out of bed on 3 consecutive days. Average the 3, and take that to be your resting heart rate. Here's the rest of the equation:

1. Subtract your age from 220 to get your predicted maximum heart rate (MHR).

2. Subtract your resting heart rate (RHR) from your MHR.

3. Multiply that number by 60 percent and also 85 percent.

4. Add your RHR to each of these values for the low end and high end of your target heart-rate zone.

Bar Talk

Your **target heart rate** is the most efficient zone within which you gain a significant cardiovascular benefit from your aerobic exercise.

Sounds complicated but it's not. For example: Deidre Johnson-Cane, age 42; resting heart rate, 72. Here's how she would figure out her target heart rate:

1. 220 − 42 = 178
2. 178 − 72 = 106
3. 106 × .60 = 63.6
4. 72 + 63.6 = **136**

So Deidre's target heart rate is 136.

How to Measure

You can take your pulse in two locations: your radial pulse is on the thumb side of your wrist; your carotid pulse is on your neck on either side of your throat. Use your index and middle finger to check your pulse at either site.

Weight a Minute

If you take your pulse at your carotid artery, be sure not to press too hard. It only takes a light touch. Too much pressure on the artery can result in a sudden decrease in blood pressure. We don't want you fainting in the middle of a workout.

Once you find your pulse, count the first beat you feel as 0, the next as 1, then 2, and so on, for 10 seconds. Multiply that figure by 6 to get your heart rate in beats per minute.

If you find that your pulse is ticking along comfortably at 138 beats per minute, say 5 beats or so above your calculated target heart rate, keep going. If, however, you're unable to mutter your name three consecutive times, slow down until you can tell someone what you had for dinner last night. In other words, use common sense. Jonathan recently saw a new gym member running on a treadmill like a businessman sprinting for the last train home. It seemed like only a matter of minutes before he was expelled from the revolving belt like a watermelon seed squeezed from one's fingers. When Jonathan asked this ambitious but misguided chap what he was doing, the wheezing runner explained that he was 5 beats below his target zone. (Jonathan checked his pulse and found out that in fact he was over his target zone by a wide margin.)

The moral of this story: check your heart rate a few times to get an accurate reading.

Second, listen to your body. Target heart rates are good guides, but they're not written in stone. If you're cruising along comfortably at the top end of your zone, that's fine. If on the other hand, you're struggling to keep pace at the low end of the zone, it's okay to back off a little.

If you don't want to be bothered with taking your pulse but want to be sure you're training in your target zone, check out a heart-rate monitor. With a wireless transmission sent from a chest strap to a wristwatch receiver, you get an accurate reading of your heart rate. Some treadmills, bikes, and stair climbers in your gym may also be able to read your heart rate directly from the transmitter. Polar is the best known and most widely used heart-rate monitor manufacturer, though others, including Cardiosport, have entered the market. Models range from the simplest version, which tells you nothing but your heart rate, to ones with alarms to tell you when you're out of your training zone, to the real fancy-schmancy ones with a stopwatch, bicycle speedometer, and computer interface.

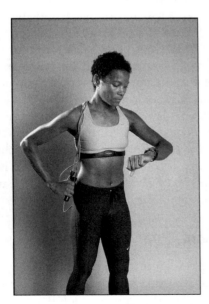

A heart-rate monitor is an effective training tool.

(Photo courtesy of Polar)

Take a Class

Within the gym, there are numerous ways to exercise aerobically. Before former martial arts standout Billy Blanks made Tae Bo a national exercise rage, the craze was spinning. Before that, there were step classes and aerobic dance.

Some people look at these theme classes as gimmicky—and we suppose some of them are—but many are great ways to churn and burn in a group setting. The workouts can be quite demanding, but the group dynamic and pulsating music distract you from the intensity of your effort. Even if you're highly motivated and work out diligently on your own, taking a class is a fun way to diversify your routine. If you're someone who needs to be motivated, these classes may be just what you need.

Spot Me

Exercises that use large muscle groups like your legs are usually your best bet for cardiovascular exercise. It's much easier and more comfortable to elevate your heart rate when using your legs, or legs and arms together, than when using just your arms.

In the following sections, we discuss briefly the various forms of aerobic activities available in a majority of gyms.

Spinning Out

Spinning, which is done on an exercise bike, was developed in California by a character named Johnny G. Typically accompanied by loud, funky tunes and sparkling and flashing lights, you stand and sit, spinning fast and slow to the calls of your instructor. No one moves (at least not forward), but you get an incredible workout. Because each rider adjusts the tension on his or her own bike, spinning can accommodate a diverse group of participants.

In case you think spinning is just for Jane Fonda types, here's an interesting case study: One winter, rather than fighting the nasty New York winter, Jonathan and several of his cycling teammates regularly took spinning classes with cyclist Kirk Whiteman, a former world champion sprinter whose thighs resemble oak trees. If their early season race results were any indication, those wintertime sweat-fests did the trick.

Flash Dance

Aerobic dance has been a mainstay of health club aerobics and home exercise tapes for many years. Ranging from high impact (lots of jumping) to low impact (no jumping), a good aerobics class is a fun way to work your upper and lower body. Like spin classes, the instructor cranks the tunes and tries to motivate participants to push a bit harder than they could push themselves. However, the good teachers make sure you're working at a pace comfortable for you. Some classes emphasize choreography and fancy moves and end up being more style than substance. Be sure the class is led by a nationally certified instructor—not a dancer.

> **Weight a Minute**
>
> Many of the early aerobic dance tapes and classes contained countless contraindicated movements. In fact, they're not perfect today, either. Look for classes and tapes taught by certified instructors—not dancers.

About 10 years ago, another variation of the basic aerobics classes, called step aerobics, hit the scene. This class uses a step that you hop up and down on to get your heart rate up. You can choose from two step heights; the higher the step, the more intense the exercise.

One of the temptations when you first take one of these classes is to try to keep up with the Joneses. Resist that urge, and go at your own pace. Often the pace of the class is just too fast, even if you've been running and working out with weights. If you find you're huffing and puffing so hard you're thinking about pulling the fire alarm, throttle back. Don't just stop. This will cause blood to pool in your legs. Instead, alter your movements. For example, if the instructor wants jumping, instead you can hop from side to side at a comfortable pace.

The second important thing to remember is hydration, hydration, and hydration! You should drink 8 to 16 ounces of water 30 to 60 minutes before exercise, 4 to 10 ounces of water every 15 minutes during your workout, and 8 to 16 ounces of water after exercise. Doing strenuous exercise in a hot, smallish room will have you sweating like you're in a sauna.

As we've pointed out many times, exercising without proper hydration is like moving lead weight. Take it from Deidre, who for some reason has shunned drinking pure water for most of her life. (She's happy to drink coffee, soda, or juice, but the pure stuff isn't her cup of tea.) Even though she drinks more water now, she forgets some days. When this happens, she can be on a modest 5-mile run and suddenly feel as if she's slogging through mud. Her breathing becomes labored, and her concentration is shot. *Why do I feel so awful?* she wonders, until it hits her like a waterfall—*drats, forgot the water.*

Run, Spot, Run

Running is as pure a sport as you can get. All you need is a good pair of sneakers, shorts, and a T-shirt. (For the women, a jog bra is usually a plus.) The beauty of running is its versatility: if you're feeling solitary, boom, you're out the door alone with your thoughts. If you want company, it's easy to find a mate eager to join you. If you don't know anyone who likes to run, joining a running club is an easy way to find a partner.

When you start out, it's important to learn how to pace yourself so you can cover the distance you set out to run. To lose weight, running at a conversational pace for 30 to 40 minutes is more important than how many miles you go. For cardiovascular fitness, it's helpful to know exactly how far you're running so you can measure your times as you continue to train. Again, for particular training tips, joining a running club is a great way to go. Typically, clubs have "speed" days at a track as well as long-distance days. If there's not a club in your area, check out one of the many books dedicated to the subject. *Runner's World* magazine also is a good guide to training tips and local races in your town or city.

![hand pointing icon] **Flex Facts**

Runner's World is a great resource for training tips as well as a list of local races in your city or town. Prefer to surf the web? Check www.active.com or www.coolrunning.com for up-to-date calendars.

Step, Two, Three, Four ...

Step machines such as the StairMaster offer another great aerobic workout. Essentially, all you're doing is walking up and down on a pair of pedals. You set the level of intensity and time and start stepping. While this is a very simple exercise, we often see people using the machine with their arms fully extended on the handrails bearing a lot of their weight. Clearly, this makes the exercise much easier to perform and much less effective—roughly the equivalent of hanging from a bar and placing your tippy-toes on a scale. If you need to lock out your elbows while you're doing your thing, lessen the intensity.

Cheating in this fashion not only guarantees that your workout will be compromised, but you also won't burn as many calories as the machine's console says you do.

Jonathan's personal favorite step machine is the Gauntlet. The Gauntlet, made by Stair-Master, is basically a set of revolving steps that enables you to actually mimic climbing stairs as opposed to the up-and-down movement on most other step equipment. More than anything else, it's like walking up a down escalator (a training method that once got Jonathan severely reprimanded by a perplexed guard during his college days). When training for the race up the Empire State Building, Jonathan has been known to spend 2 or 3 hours on a Gauntlet. For those of you with slightly saner aspirations, 20 to 30 minutes will suffice.

One of the good features of these machines is the feedback they offer. Almost all step equipment has a computer pad that enables you to work out to several different programs. You can do a steady climb, a hill workout, and various permutations in between. These various programs offer a good change of pace for those of you who get bored doing the same thing all the time.

Some pieces of equipment also take your pulse as you hold the side rails. This is convenient because you don't have to find and hold your pulse while watching the clock. It also saves you the burdensome task of having to multiply lofty sums like 24 times 6.

The Least You Need to Know

- If you want to get strong, lift weights; if you want to be truly fit, don't neglect the treadmill.

- You can figure out how hard to do your cardiovascular work in one of two ways: the talk test or monitoring your heart rate.

- Spinning, stair climbers, and aerobics classes are some of the best indoor cardiovascular workouts you'll find at your gym.

In This Chapter

- ◆ Eliminating the excuses
- ◆ Making the time to work out
- ◆ Planning is the key
- ◆ Getting social: the social side of working out

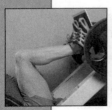
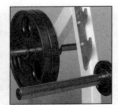
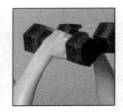
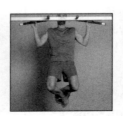
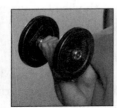
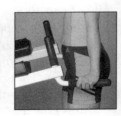

Chapter 20

Hurry Up and Weight

Okay, let's assume you've read our persuasive prose in the previous 19 chapters and we've finally convinced you there are sound reasons why you *should* lift; the concern you might have now is that you're not sure if you *can*. Fret not! The old saying, "Where there's a will, there's a way" is especially true when it comes to exercise. In this chapter, we help you rid yourself of all the usual excuses so you can get on the road to fitness.

It's Easier Than You Think

First off, working out effectively (and efficiently) is easier and far less time-consuming than you may think—if you know what you're doing. You can get a great and thorough workout in 30 or 45 minutes. Sound skimpy? Do each set to failure (to the point you can't do one more) and you'll leave the gym so exhausted (and well trained) you'll be unable to lift anything heavier than a tofu sandwich for a while.

Like we said, if time is an issue and you're unable to work out as often as you'd like, you need not despair. You can fit working out into your lifestyle. For instance, if you live a reasonable distance from your place of business, you can walk to work instead of driving. (Just for the record, 70-year-old former running great Ted Corbett walks 11 miles from his home in the Bronx to work in Manhattan each day.) Similarly, if you work in an office building, you can motor up the steps instead of using the elevator. Not only will you be stretching your legs and improving your cardiovascular fitness, but you're likely to earn a reputation as "the fitness nut."

The main point to keep in mind is that nothing has power over your training unless you give it power. In other words, take stock of the excuses you manufacture, and gently toss them where they belong: the garbage heap. We all do it, but the ability to generate excuses—the "my piranha ate my gym shorts" kind of thing—has more to do with fear, sloth, or some other mental block than it does with an insurmountable obstacle.

Just for fun, let's look at the "Top 10 Lame Excuses Not to Exercise" we've heard:

1. "I forgot my socks."
2. "My dog ate my membership card."
3. "I'm having a bad hair day."
4. "My tattoo is drying."
5. "I just did my nails."
6. "My outfit doesn't match."
7. "I'm premenstrual."
8. "My allergies are acting up."
9. "I don't have time; happy hour will be over soon."
10. "I'm hung over."

A few of the honorable mentions include: "I had a fight with my girlfriend/boyfriend," "My cat died," and "I got some Ben Gay in my eye." Those feeble lines are easy to debunk, but let's take a quick look at the top five excuses that carry a bit more weight:

1. **"I'm too busy."** Good solid excuse. However, consider the triathlete Joe often trains with, a 50-year-old architect we'll call Frank L. Wright. Mr. Wright works at his job at least 40 to 60 hours a week, yet has qualified for 3 Hawaii Ironman triathlons, run more than 25 marathons, and trains as many as 30 hours a week, including 3 weight-lifting sessions a week. Okay, so he's a training freak. The point is that if he can work and exercise that much, you can manage to work out 2 to 4 hours a week. It's all a question of desire and time management.

2. **"I'm too tired."** Not bad! But ironically (or not), most of the time exercising will revive you, turning a groggy, cranky human into a more delightful version of your prestressed self. Being flexible helps. If you're feeling weary, you can just lighten the load and lift less strenuously. Sometimes a good warm-up will turn you around. If not, just breathing deeply for the time you lift will do wonders for you.

3. **"Gyms are too expensive."** Remember that a gym doesn't have to be expensive at all: there are a wide variety of fees and even many ways to work out without a gym.

4. **"My back, neck, wrist, shoulder, knee hurts."** Stressing an injured body part is plain stupid. However, there are many ways to work out with your injury and as many exercises to help injured body parts mend faster. An example of the former occurred when Joe broke his wrist while training for the Boston Marathon. Not only did he continue to run (no problem there), he continued doing strength-training exercises on his noninjured side. (Studies show that exercising the uninjured or contralateral [opposite] side speeds recovery.)

5. **"It takes too long."** Sorry! As we've said, not only can you make biking, walking, skating, or running part of your daily transportation, you can make terrific strength-training gains by spending as little as 90 minutes to 2 hours a week lifting weights at home or at the gym.

Now that we've got the excuses out of the way, read on to discover the workout options available to even the busiest multitaskers.

Working Out Before Work

A few years back, Joe took a Navy SEAL training course for 2 weeks as research for an article he was writing for the *New York Times*. A notorious slow starter in the morning, Joe grimaced at the thought of exercising at 5 A.M. in Manhattan's Central Park. What he realized, other than the fact that homeless men do their most productive collecting between 4 and 6 A.M., is that working out early gets the day off to a flying start and affords an expansiveness that is likely to leave you feeling downright giddy. In fact, Joe felt so virtuous that when he'd finished at 6:45 A.M., he shouted "Slackers!" at the joggers and cyclists circling the park in the cool of the morning for getting such a "late" start.

Weight a Minute

If you're planning to go for a run or bike ride at dawn, be sure you've chosen a safe route. And in the darker winter months, it's a good idea to wear a reflective vest.

Clearly, getting out of bed early to get to the gym or park requires some good solid willpower. However, once you make it a part of your daily routine, you'll start to get cranky if you're unable to start your day with an endorphin rush. To quote that old adage: "One hour in the morning is worth three in the afternoon." (Just for the record: it typically takes about 8 weeks to establish a routine as a habit.)

Getting an early start requires some organizational skills. One of the guys in Joe's Navy SEAL class, a Wall Street trader who had to go from Central Park to his office, ran through the park schlepping a garment bag over his shoulder. He looked like a complete goof, but we have to admire his dedication.

Although that particular exercise predicament may not apply to you, some people are resistant to the morning workout simply because they don't know what to do with their gear—sweaty clothes, towels, beauty aids—when they go from the gym straight to work. If that's the case, invest in a rental locker at the gym where you can store your accoutrements.

Flex Facts

Americans spend 2,300 hours in front of the television set every year; researchers report that the average family member now spends more than 7 hours a day watching television and 14 minutes a day talking to other family members. We're asking you to devote 75 to 100 hours a year to lifting.

The Lunch Break Plan

If, however, waking at the crack of dawn is as appealing as getting pecked to death by ducks, consider working out during lunch. For this strategy to be effective, your gym needs to be within shouting distance of your workplace. If you have to travel far to get there, you'll end up frittering away much of your exercise time.

Unless you live in a country that recognizes a daily *ciesta*, don't plan on going hog wild at lunch. Remember, you've got to change into your workout gear, pump iron, shower, and change back into your grownup clothes—so plan your routine accordingly so it won't have you rushing through your workout like a bike messenger through Manhattan. Working out under duress can turn a stress-buster into a stress-inducer and often leads to injury because you're more focused on finishing than being mindful about using proper form.

"But it's lunchtime," you say. What about that deli around the corner that whispers your name? Well, call us austere, but here's a good way to approach the midday meal: first, eat a large, healthful breakfast (a mixture of protein and carbs to avoid that coffee-and-donut, late-morning crash), then snack on a piece of fruit and/or some nuts an hour or two before noon. This way, by the time lunchtime rolls around, you've kept your blood-sugar level elevated and won't be ready to gnaw on the pencil sharpener. (Having a low sugar level is the reason we become hungry.) After your workout, eat a sandwich, a piece of fruit, or a cup of yogurt at your desk. This combination of protein, carbs, and fat should fill you up without the threat of you curling up for a nap under your desk.

Finally, working out during the day may give you more energy and incentive to work a bit harder and more effectively at your job. This increased productivity may even get you a raise. But beware—a promotion may lead to more responsibility, and that could crimp your midday power workout!

Spot Me

Before you go to the gym, eat yogurt, a piece of fruit, or some nuts, which will provide you with some prework-out energy. For lunch, try a turkey, lettuce, and tomato sandwich with mustard on whole-wheat bread. The combination of carbohydrates and protein prevents fatigue, the mustard is less fattening than mayo, and whole-wheat bread is more nutritious than the white stuff.

Work Out Postwork

The most popular time to work out is after work. While scores of your cronies saunter up to the corner bar, you'll be loading iron onto another kind of bar—one that will leave you without a headache or a cash deficit.

Let's look at the pluses of working out after work:

◆ You'll have more time to do a thorough workout.

◆ It's a fine time to schmooze with the workout set.

◆ You'll head home feeling refreshed after a long day at the office.

◆ You're less likely to kick the dog or quarrel with your mate.

That's the good news; the bad news about an after-work workout includes the following:

◆ A crowded gym can be a tough place to get a good workout. Unless your facility is spacious and well equipped, you might have to wait for a particular apparatus (bad for the flow) and/or be rushed off the station you're using. (We give you some strategies for how to deal with this later.)

◆ Too much chatting. It's one thing to be social and another to try to work out at a cocktail party. If you're trying to work out efficiently, it can be disconcerting when someone is telling you the latest "good news/bad news" joke. Sure, your repertoire of bad jokes may increase, but you may find yourself barely breaking a sweat.

The fact is, the hardest part of working out is getting to the gym. The "just take the day off" devil sitting on your shoulder is a loud and divisive force, especially if you've had a hard day at work.

Clearly it's important to listen to the rhythms and whims of your body—exercise is, after all, supposed to enhance your life, not turn you into a guilt-ridden mess. (Always remember: a fitness regimen is not punishment for a flawed body, but a way to enhance your natural gifts.)

Keep in mind that the fatigue you're feeling is usually all in your head. After a few minutes of working out, you're likely to get your second wind. When this happens, you'll be glad you exercised your willpower as well as your body. As fitness expert Steve Ilg writes, "You are developing inner strength in addition to outer strength." Put another way, Shakespeare said: "Our bodies are our gardens, to which our wills are gardeners."

Just to show you what's possible if you're really motivated, consider Joe's Ironman architect friend who typically runs before work, swims at lunch, and cycles after work. Although he might not have the world's most exciting social life, he does shower more than a supermodel and gets to consume more calories than your average circus elephant.

Let's Get Ready for the Weekend!

Working out is generally easier on the weekends than during the week for the simple reason that most of us have more free time on those precious 2 days. However, it's also far too easy to fritter away your workout time when you have the whole day stretching out in front of you. That's why it's a good idea to "schedule" your exercise for an hour or two the day before so you have a plan—and then stick to it.

If family responsibilities present a conflict, do what we suggested in the preceding text. Either get up early and squeeze in a workout while the toddler is still asleep (you'll need someone to watch the snoozer, of course), or schedule your exercise for late in the afternoon just before you plan to paint the town red. We know a lot of city dwellers who follow this weekend ritual: a late afternoon nap, work out at the gym, light dinner, and then it's party time.

Depending on the location of your gym, the weekend workout can get tricky. If you both work and live near your institution of higher fitness, you're fine. If you have to travel very far from home to the gym, on the other hand, you might want to make the trip more utilitarian by running errands en route. If the weather is good and you're not pressed for time, cycling to the gym is a great way to warm up and burn some extra calories. Regardless, keep the gym's distance from home as well as from your workplace in mind when you purchase your gym membership. If it's possible to find one located relatively equidistant from both, that's the way to go. Another approach is to consider joining a gym that's part of a chain so you can work out at any of its affiliated gyms. That way, at home, at work, or even on the road, you've got your endorphins covered.

You Brush Your Teeth, Don't You?

A woman named Lady Mary Wortley Montagu once said: "The trick is to die young as late as possible." Working out is a time-honored way to accomplish this noble aim.

By now we hope we've convinced you that not only *should* you work out, you *need* to work out. Most civilized people find the time every day to eat, bathe, and brush their teeth. Similarly, working out should become a standard part of your daily (or almost-daily) health maintenance program.

Weight training may not make you live longer, but it will help ensure you live better. Your muscles, connective tissue, and bones will get stronger; you'll have more energy, coordination, agility, and *savoir faire*. (Okay, the last one is debatable, but it sounds good and French lifters claim this as an added benefit.)

For all these reasons and more, thinking about working out not as a negotiable option but as something that is necessary for your general health and well-being should help get you off your duff and into action.

> **Flex Facts**
>
> Dr. Urho M. Kajala of the University of Helsinki tracked 16,000 healthy sets of twins for an average of 19 years. Those twins who exercised regularly—taking half-hour walks just twice a week—cut their risk of death by 44 percent. Even occasional exercisers were 30 percent less likely to die young than were their control group (sedentary) twins.

Sweat Socially

The gym is a great equalizer: status, wealth, and social airs are generally tossed out the window because the assembled crowd—corporate bigwigs, bus drivers, unemployed actors, teachers—sweat under one roof in shorts, spandex, and T-shirts. (It's hard to take even a dignified CEO seriously when he's walking around with a sweaty crotch.)

Sure, the muscleheads flex in the mirror and beauty queens sashay around the room, but just about everyone in attendance is there for similar reasons that serve to unite us.

Although each gym is different, in general the social dynamics in a gym are amusing: a curious combination of neighborhood watering hole, soap-opera set, and endorphin commune. You'll be able to discuss the big game, mourn the stock market losses, hear about the latest movie, and dish the dating gossip. But unlike a bar or party where there's a premium placed on "making a connection," the gym is a lower-pressure conversation zone—the best of both worlds. You can chat if you like or remain mum and pump iron with a purpose.

> **Flex Facts**
>
> Six months after the start of a fitness program for Dallas police officers, officer commendations jumped 39 percent, while the amount of sick leave taken by exercising officers dropped 29 percent. Such statistics only confirm the integral relationship between mind, body, and spirit. If this sounds like New Age mumbo-jumbo, ask the Dallas cops about their regimen. Better yet, work out and see for yourself.

We've worked out next to people for years and never done more than bat an eye in their direction; other gym rats become fast and lasting friends. And we've peacefully coexisted silently next to familiar faces only to find out one day that they are excellent company. That's part of the fun about hanging out in a place filled with aspiration.

Way back when, Deidre and Jonathan met at the Hunter College gym. And Joe and Deidre met at their gym in Brooklyn. The three of us are quite serious about working out—heck, Deidre can *deadlift* a compact car and has won two World Powerlifting titles—but when you encounter a smiling face, you just can't help but schmooze. Before you know it, you're part of a healthy subculture—a fitness cult!

It's interesting to note that more and more businesses are finding that a healthy and relaxed employee is a more productive employee and an employee who is less likely to take sick days. That's why corporate fitness centers are appearing all over the country. If your company provides an on-site gym (or has a contract with one nearby), run—don't walk—there ASAP. Many are free (or modestly priced) and often offer payroll deductions so you never have to think about paying your gym bill. Furthermore, these facilities tend to be spiffy—stocked with all the amenities to leave you looking and smelling like a rose.

The Least You Need to Know

◆ It's important to try not to fall prey to excuses that keep you from meeting your fitness goals.

◆ Choose your workout time with care; you have plenty of options: before work, at lunch, after work, and on weekends.

◆ View working out not as an option or a hardship, but instead as a joyous and necessary part of life's journey.

◆ Joining a gym just might expand your social life—if you want it to.

In This Chapter

◆ Maintaining muscles with resistance bands

◆ Choosing your weapon

◆ Working out with bands: eight great exercises

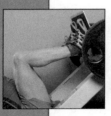
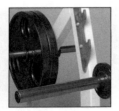
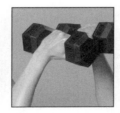
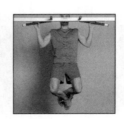
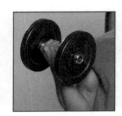
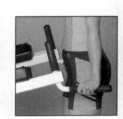

Chapter 21

Bands on the Run

Freeweights or machines are the most conventional and efficient way to strengthen your muscles, but you can't always get to the gym to use them. If you're on the road, stuck at work, or for any other reason you can't make it to the gym, you don't have to miss your workout altogether.

In Deidre's physical therapy office, they're known as Therabands. At her gym, they go by Dynabands. Generically, they're called resistance bands. A rose is a rose is a rose, and a resistance band is basically a giant rubber band on steroids. They're color coded according to their level of resistance and can be cut to any length for use in a variety of exercises. Using resistance bands as your sole (or even main) source of strength training won't get you entered in a powerlifting meet any time soon, nor can you adequately address all the muscles you might want to, but it is a safe, inexpensive, easy way to maintain strength when a gym workout is impractical.

To weigh the resistance bands pros and cons …

Pros of Resistance Bands

◆ Easy to pack.

◆ Variable resistance. (They come in different grades, and you can pull them looser or tighter.)

◆ Can be used for a variety of exercises.

◆ Safe.

Cons of Resistance Bands

◆ Resistance is not constant throughout the full range of motion. (It's fairly easy at first and gets harder as you pull it tighter.)

◆ Although effective for some smaller muscle groups, bands are not as useful for larger ones such as your glutes, quads, and hamstrings, where greater resistance is needed.

◆ They break. Stretch the bands enough times, and they'll wear out.

Spot Me

The best things about resistance bands is that they're so easily portable and easy to use when you're on the road (or even in your office if you can't make it to the gym). We're not saying you'll get in great shape using them exclusively, but their convenience and ease of use makes them a practical way to maintain fitness when a visit to the gym is impossible.

The trick to using resistance bands is to choose a band with the appropriate amount of resistance and to have some tension on the band as you start the exercise. Having some tension means your muscles are firing even at the beginning of the range of motion. If you're in need of a real challenge, you can always fold the band over or use more than one at a time to make the exercise particularly difficult.

Flex Facts

Because bands gain tension as they're stretched, their resistance level changes throughout the range of motion. You'll find that exercises are easier at the beginning and harder at the end of the movement. To ensure benefit throughout the ROM, start the exercise with some tension on the band.

Let's take a look at some of our favorite band exercises.

Band Low Row

The band low row simulates the low cable row, working the muscles of your back and biceps. Here's the drill:

1. Sit on the floor and wrap the band around the balls of your feet.
2. With elbows bent, pull your arms back while squeezing your shoulder blades together.
3. Slowly return to the starting position.

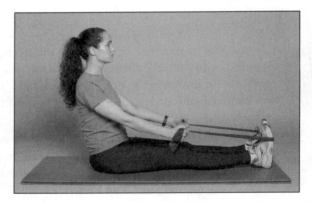

Band low row start/finish position.

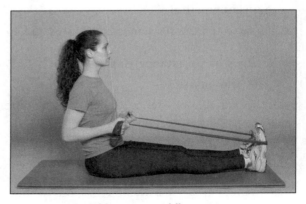

Band low row middle position.

Band Chest Press

When you can't make it to the gym, this is a great alternate to the bench press. Here's how to properly perform the exercise:

1. Wrap the band around your back.
2. Grip the ends of the band with both hands.
3. Press your arms forward, bringing them together at the end.
4. Slowly return to the starting position.

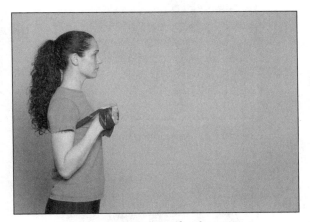

Band chest press start/finish position.

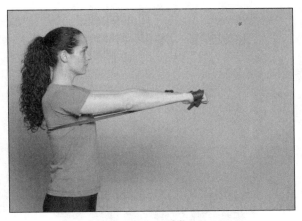

Band chest press middle position.

Band Lateral Raise

The band lateral raise is an effective alternate to the freeweight version. Here's what you need to know:

1. Stand with your feet shoulder-width apart, and step on the middle of the band.
2. Hold one end of the band in each hand.
3. Maintaining a slight bend in each elbow, slowly raise your arms to the side until they reach shoulder height.
4. Slowly return to the starting position.

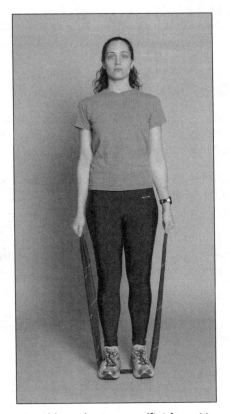

Band lateral raise start/finish position.

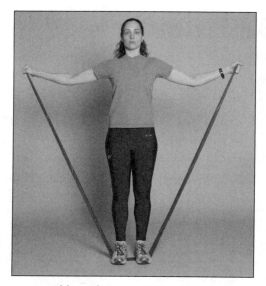

Band lateral raise middle position.

Band Front Raise

Front raises with a resistance band are quite effective in isolating the anterior part of your deltoid. Here's how to do them properly:

1. Stand with your feet shoulder-width apart, and step on the band.
2. Hold one end of the band in one hand.
3. While maintaining proper alignment, slowly raise your arms in front of you until your reach shoulder height.
4. Slowly return to the starting position.

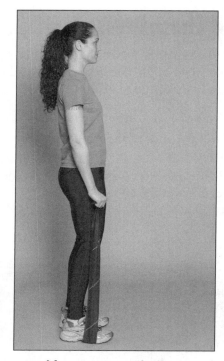

Band front raise start/finish position.

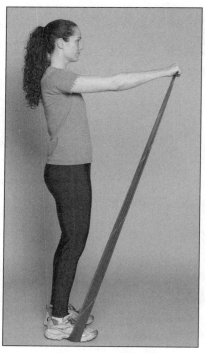

Band front raise middle position.

Band Biceps Curls

You probably won't make it to Muscle Beach with just bands, but using them for biceps curls will work in a pinch. Here's how to do them right:

1. Stand with your feet shoulder-width apart.
2. Hold each end of the band and stand on the middle of it.
3. Ensure that there's some tension on the band in the starting position, wrapping it around your hand if necessary.
4. Slowly curl your hands to your shoulder by bending your elbow.
5. Return to the starting position in a slow, controlled fashion.

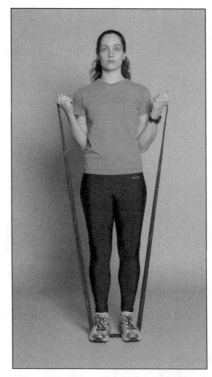

Band biceps curl middle position.

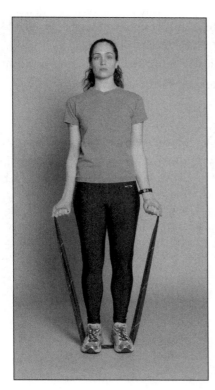

Band biceps curl start/finish position.

Band Triceps Extension

Once you've worked your biceps, you always want to train the opposite side of your arm—the triceps. This is what you need to know:

1. Grasp each end of the band with your hands.
2. Hold the nonexercising hand at your side.
3. Bring the exercising hand behind your head, near your opposite shoulder.
4. Keeping your upper arm vertical, raise your exercising hand by straightening your elbow.
5. Slowly return to the starting position.
6. Repeat on the other side.

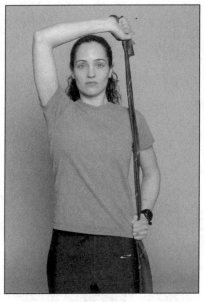

Band triceps extension start/finish
position.

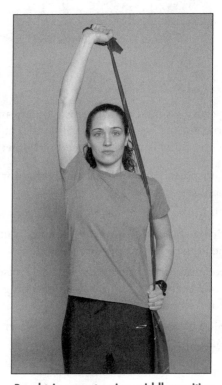

Band triceps extension middle position.

Band Internal Rotation

Bands are very effective for internal and external rotation exercises. While these are not flashy or exciting exercises, they are great for working the muscles of your rotator cuff and are, therefore, valuable for any athlete who plays racquet or throwing sports. Here are the basics:

1. Securely tie a band around a stable, waist-high object such as a door knob.
2. Stand with the band at your side.
3. Grasp the end of the band with the hand closest to the secured end.
4. Bend your elbow to 90 degrees, and rotate your arm outward.
5. Keeping your elbow pinned against your torso and your shoulders squared, slowly rotate your arm inward.
6. Slowly return to the starting position.
7. Repeat on the other side.

Spot Me

Bands are not our preferred method of resistance for most exercises, but they're perfect for internal and external rotation. Using dumbbells requires you to lay in uncomfortable positions and doesn't allow for tension through the full range of motion, but bands are easy to use in any position.

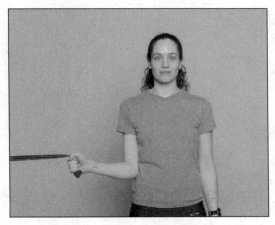

Band internal rotation start/finish position.

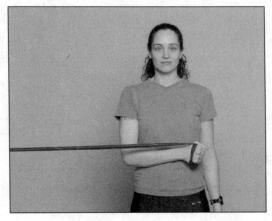

Band internal rotation middle position.

Band External Rotation

External rotation is the kissin' cousin to internal rotation. It, too, is a great rotator cuff exercise. Here's what to do:

1. Securely tie a band around a stable, waist-high object such as a door knob.
2. Stand with the band at your side.
3. Grasp the end of the band with the hand farthest from the secured end.
4. Bend your elbow to 90 degrees, and rotate your arm inward.

5. Keeping your elbow pinned against your torso and your shoulders squared, slowly rotate your arm outward.
6. Slowly return to the starting position.
7. Repeat on the other side.

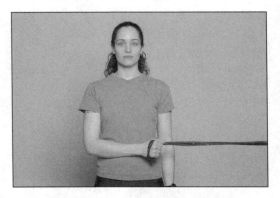

Band internal rotation start/finish position.

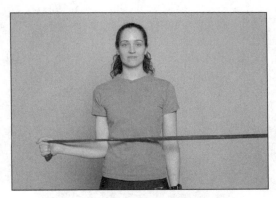

Band internal rotation middle position.

The Least You Need to Know

◆ Resistance bands are a viable alternative when you're traveling or otherwise unable to make it to the gym.

◆ Choose the appropriate level of resistance when picking your band.

◆ Ensure that there's tension on the band at the start, so your muscle is worked through the full range of motion.

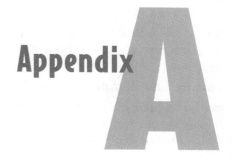

Appendix

Glossary

abdominals (abs)   Muscles of the midsection.

abduction   Sideways movement away from the body.

abductors   Muscles that move your leg away from your body.

adduction   Sideways movement in the direction toward the body.

adductors   Muscles that draw your leg in toward your body from an outward position.

aerobic   Exercise that requires a significant and sustained supply of oxygen. Literally means "in the presence of oxygen."

alternating grip (reverse grip)   A grip with which you hold the bar with the fingers of one hand facing your body (pronated) and the fingers of the other hand facing away from your body (supinated).

amino acids   The structural material or "building blocks" of protein.

anaerobic   Exercise that can take place in the absence of oxygen.

anterior   The front of the body.

assisted reps   Repetitions performed with the help of a spotter.

atrophy   The loss of size of a muscle. The opposite of hypertrophy.

barbell   A straight freeweight on which plates can be added for increased resistance.

bench press   A power-lifting exercise that involves lying on your back and pushing a weight from your chest.

biceps   The muscle in the front of the upper arm, responsible for bending (flexing) the elbow.

breakdowns A technique in which once you fatigue, you decrease the weight being used and do a few extra reps.

bursa A padlike sac that acts to reduce friction between tendon and bone or tendon and ligament.

bursitis Inflammation of the bursa.

cardiovascular exercise Any activity that improves your cardiovascular system. Your body's cardiovascular system includes your heart, lungs, and circulatory system.

carpal tunnel syndrome A condition that is often caused by repetitive activities done with improper body mechanics, such as typing with your wrists in an extended position, or repetitive squeezing activities. The median nerve swells and is unable to pass comfortably through the small bones in your wrist (carpals). Symptoms of carpal tunnel syndrome are numbness, tingling, or a sharp, shooting pain into your hand.

clean and jerk An Olympic weight-lifting exercise in which the lifter hoists the weight from the platform to the shoulders in one motion (clean) and then thrusts the bar from his or her shoulders to an overhead position in one motion while splitting his or her legs (jerk).

collar A safety device that helps secure plates on a barbell.

compound movement An exercise, such as the bench press, squat, or lat pull-down, that involves the movement of more than one joint at a time.

concentric contraction The shortening of a muscle as it exerts force.

contract Literally speaking, to draw together or shorten. When contracted, a muscle shortens and produces movement.

contracture A condition in which a joint (shoulder, elbow, wrist, finger, hip, knee, or ankle) is unable to be fully straightened or fully bent.

deadlift A powerlifting maneuver in which the weighted bar is on the floor, the lifter bends his or her knees and hips to reach the bar, and then lifts it to midthigh.

delayed onset muscle soreness (DOMS) The temporary, post-workout pain you feel in your muscles usually within 24 hours of your workout, which peaks after 48 hours.

deltoid Major muscle of the shoulder. Divided into medial, posterior, and anterior sections.

diaphragm A muscle used in respiration.

dumbbell A handheld freeweight.

eccentric contraction A lengthening of the muscle as it exerts force but is overcome by the resistance.

erector spinae Muscles of the back that run along the spine.

ergogenic aid Any product that improves athletic or physical performance.

extend To increase the angle between body parts, as in straightening the elbow or knee.

fast-twitch muscle fiber A powerful, easily fatigued muscle fiber.

female athletic triad A phenomenon common among competitive female athletes that consists of eating disorders, amenorrhea (absence of the menstrual flow), and osteoporosis.

flex To decrease the angle between body parts, as in bending the elbow or knee. (Commonly, but incorrectly, used to refer to contracting a muscle.)

freeweight A handheld weight, such as a barbell or dumbbell.

gastrocnemius A muscle in the back of the lower leg, responsible for raising the heel over the toe, especially when the knee is straight.

gluteus (glutes) The gluteus maximus (the gluteus medius and gluteus minimus are much smaller and weaker), responsible for extension of the hip.

hamstrings   Muscles in the back of the upper leg, responsible for bending the knee and extending the hip. Made up of the biceps femoris, semitendinosus, and semimembranosus muscles.

hyperextend   To extend a joint beyond straight.

hyperplasia   An increase in the amount of muscle fibers in some animals. Does not appear to occur in humans.

hypertrophy   The growth of a muscle and the individual fibers that make it up. This growth usually occurs as a result of an external stimulus such as weight lifting.

impingement   The pinching or squeezing of the internal structures of the shoulder (tendons of the rotator cuff, bursa, ligaments, and nerves). This pinching causes pain on elevation of the arm.

isolation exercise   A lift that uses only one joint and, therefore, focuses on one muscle.

isometric contraction   A muscle action that results in no movement because the muscle force and the resistance are equal.

lactic acid   Byproduct of anaerobic work that causes fatigue and a burning sensation.

latissimus dorsi (lats)   The large, fan-shaped muscles of the middle and upper back.

ligaments   The connective tissue between bones.

lordosis   The natural inward curve of the lumbar or lower spine.

muscle pull   *See* muscle strain.

muscle strain   A trauma to the muscle or tendon caused by excessive contraction or stretching.

negatives   An advanced technique in which you stress the eccentric phase of an exercise.

Olympic weight lifting   A competitive sport that includes the snatch and the clean and jerk.

overtraining   A phenomenon that occurs when you exercise excessively without allowing sufficient recovery between workouts.

palpitations   An abnormally rapid throbbing or fluttering of the heart.

pectorals (pecs)   The large muscles in the chest.

phlebitis   An inflammation of a vein.

plates   Weighted discs added to a bar to increase its weight. Plates most often come in denominations of 2½, 5, 10, 25, 35, and 45 pounds.

plyometrics   Controversial exercises that use bounding techniques to build "explosive" power.

posing   A facet of bodybuilding in which the competitor demonstrates his or her physical assets by assuming various positions that show off his or her muscularity and proportion.

posterior   The rear of the body.

powerlifting   A competitive sport that includes the squat, bench press, and deadlift.

pronation   Turning the hand so the palm faces downward. Opposite of supination.

quadriceps   Muscles of the front of the upper leg, responsible for straightening the knee. Made up of the rectus femoris, vastus lateralis, vastus intermedius, and vastus medialis muscles.

range of motion (ROM)   The movement from the beginning to the finishing point of an exercise. Moving a joint from complete extension to complete flexion is considered a full range of motion.

recovery   The rest period between two sets or workouts.

repetition (rep)   The execution of an exercise one time. Consecutive repetitions are grouped into a set.

rotator cuff   Group of muscles (supraspinatus, infraspinatus, teres minor, and subscapularis) located under the deltoid.

set   A series of repetitions performed consecutively.

slow-twitch muscle fiber   A muscle fiber that has great endurance but relatively low power.

snatch   An Olympic weight-lifting exercise in which the lifter pulls the bar up from the platform. Then he or she leaps into a squat position under the bar, securing it overhead with arms held straight.

soleus   A muscle in the back of the lower leg, responsible for raising the heel over the toe, especially when the knee is bent.

specificity of training   A physiological theory that suggests that adaptations made during training depend on the type of training used.

split routine   A workout scheme in which the body is divided into different parts that are exercised on different days.

spotter   Someone who stands by to help the lifter if and when he or she can't finish a repetition. The spotter is responsible for the lifter's safety.

sprain   Damage due to overstretching of ligaments.

squat   A powerlifting maneuver that involves performing a deep-knee bend with a barbell across your back.

sticking point   A particular position during your range of motion where you have difficulty completing the repetition without assistance.

supersets   An advanced strength-training method that involves doing two exercises with no rest.

SuperSlow   A protocol that involves extremely slow movement—10 seconds for the positive phase and 5 seconds for the negative.

supination   Turning the hand so the palm faces upward. Opposite of pronation.

T cells   The cells responsible for enhancing antibody production and for killing foreign cells in the body.

target heart rate (training zone)   The desired heart-rate range to elicit a training effect while performing cardiovascular exercise.

tendinitis   A condition characterized by inflammation of a tendon.

tendon   Connective tissue that attaches muscle to bone.

trapezius (traps)   The muscle that covers the rear of the neck and shoulders.

triceps   The muscle in the back of the upper arm, responsible for straightening (extending) the elbow.

Valsalva maneuver   Holding the breath while lifting. May lead to excessive increase in blood pressure and decrease in blood returning to the heart.

VO_2 max   A measure of an individual's capacity for aerobic work. It is generally considered one of the most important factors in predicting an athlete's ability to perform in activities of more than 3 to 5 minutes.

weight belt   A thick, wide, dense leather belt used for added support for the lower back when lifting.

working in   The practice of alternating sets on a particular bench or machine with another person.

Appendix B

Resources

Aerobics and Fitness Association of America (AFAA)
15250 Ventura Boulevard, Suite 200
Sherman Oaks, CA 91403
1-877-YOURBODY (1-877-968-7263)
www.afaa.com

American College of Sports Medicine (ACSM)
PO Box 1440
Indianapolis, IN 46206-1440
317-637-9200
www.acsm.org

American Council on Exercise (ACE)
4851 Paramount Drive
San Diego, CA 92123
858-279-8227 or
1-800-825-3636
www.acefitness.org

Bowflex
2200 NE 65th Avenue
Vancouver, WA 98661
1-800-269-3539
www.bowflex.com

Concept II
105 Industrial Park Drive
Morrisville, VT 05661-9727
1-800-245-5676
www.concept2.com

Cyberpump
www.cyberpump.com

Cybex
2100 Smithtown Avenue
Ronkonkoma, NY 11779
516-585-9000
www.ecybex.com

Fitness Management
4160 Wilshire Boulevard
Los Angeles, CA 90010
323-964-4800
www.fitnessworld.com

Gatorade Sports Science Institute
617 W. Main Street
Barrington, IL 60010
1-800-616-GSSI
(1-800-616-4774)
www.gssiweb.com

Hammer Strength
2245 Gilbert Avenue
Cincinnati, OH 45206
513-221-2600
www.hammerstrength.com

Healthclubs.com
A guide to health and fitness
www.healthclubs.com

Healthfinder
U.S. Department of Health and Human Services
www.healthfinder.gov

Icarian
12660 Branford Street
Sun Valley, CA 91352
1-800-883-2421

International Health, Racquet and Sportsclub Association (IHRSA)
263 Summer Street
Boston, MA 02210
1-800-228-4772
www.ihrsa.org

LifeFitness
10601 West Belmont Avenue
Franklin Park, IL 60131
1-800-735-3867
www.lifefitness.com

Nancy Clark Sports Nutrition
www.nancyclarkrd.com

National Strength Professionals Association (NSPA)
PO Box 967
Mount Airy, MD 21771
301-829-3900 or
1-800-494-6722
www.nspainc.com

National Strength and Conditioning Association (NSCA)
3333 Landmark Circle
Lincoln, NE 68504
402-476-6669 or
1-888-746-2378
www.nsca-cc.org

Natural Strength
www.naturalstrength.com

Nautilus
709 Powerhouse Road
Independence, VA 24348-0708
1-800-NAUTILUS
(1-800-628-8458)
www.nautilus.com

Polar
1111 Marcus Avenue, Suite M15
Lake Success, NY 11042-1034
1-800-227-1314
www.polarusa.com

PowerBlock
Intellbell, Inc.
1071 32nd Avenue NW
Owatonna, MN 55060
507-451-5152
www.powerblock.com

Powerlifting USA
PO Box 467
Camarillo, CA 93011
1-800-448-7693

Soloflex
Hawthorn Farm Industrial Park
570 NE 53rd Avenue
Hillsboro, OR 97124-6494
1-800-547-8802
www.soloflex.com

StairMaster Sports
12421 Willows Road NE, Suite 100
Kirkland, WA 98034
1-800-635-2936
www.stairmaster.com

Star Trac
14410 Myford Road
Irvine, CA 92606
877-STAR-TRAC
(877-782-7872)
www.startrac.com

SuperSlow Exercise Guild
PO Box 180154
Casselberry, FL 32718-0154
407-862-2552
www.superslow.com

Total Gym
755 Arjons Drive
San Diego, CA 92126
1-800-541-4900
www.totalgym.com

Trotter
10 Trotter Way
Medway, MA 02053
1-800-677-6544

U.S. Food and Drug Administration (FDA)
5600 Fishers Lane
Rockville, MD 20857
1-888-INFO-FDA
(1-888-463-6332)
www.fda.gov

USA Powerlifting
124 West Van Buren Street
Columbia City, IN 46725
219-248-4889
www.usapowerlifting.com

USA Weightlifting
1 Olympic Plaza
Colorado Springs, CO 80909
719-866-4508
www.usaweightlifting.org

VersaClimber Heart Rate, Inc.
3190-E Airport Loop
Costa Mesa, CA 92626-2771
1-800-237-2271
www.versaclimber.com

Women's Sports Foundation
Eisenhower Park
East Meadow, NY 11554
1-800-227-3988
www.womenssportsfoundation.org

Index

T

X–Y–Z